HIGH, IT'S ME ADDICTION

HOW TO RECOGNIZE, LOVE, AND DECIDE IF YOU CAN LIVE WITH AN ADDICTED SPOUSE

DHANA RAPHAEL MICHAELS

CONTENTS

Sobriety Journal

Redeem your FREE printable copy of SOBRIETY JOURNAL
Link: https://tremendous-originator-440.ck.page/form1

INTRODUCTION

One of the most difficult things to do in the world is watch someone destroy themselves with their addiction. It's literally a tragedy in action to watch your loved one succumb to the pain that drives them to return to their addictive behaviors time and again. All you want to do is help them get better, but the truth is that you can't help them. They must make the decision to help themselves—it's an inside job, and a difficult one at that. You can support them, but the problem seems to be that you're not the most important thing in your partner's life, and thus, your influence is limited. They can't see through their addiction to see the pain they're causing their loved ones, and that's because they are genuinely ill. That illness causes them to prioritize their addiction over almost anything else in their lives, although they don't see it that way.

If you're the partner of an addict, you likely feel as though your relationship is in constant conflict. Your partner neglects your needs to the point where you have to ask yourself if they even love you. It's truly heartbreaking and an all-too-common situation. One out of every eight adults in the United States struggles with some kind of substance abuse. It's a demon that robs you of your loved one and turns them into someone entirely different from the person you once knew. The pain the addict causes themselves and their loved ones is enormous. If you're reading this book, this is something you likely already know.

For the addict, it seems there's no escaping the grasp of their habit, and indeed, addiction's steel grip on your partner's behavior lasts long after they've stopped actually enjoying the effects of their substance of choice. In their pain, they often lash out at the ones they love the most. They can be emotionally and/or physically abusive, and they're seldom logical when under the influence of their favorite substance. That can make your world seem like some kind of surrealistic horror movie with no escape. You love them; you want to help, but you, too, are powerless in the face of their addiction.

It can seem like a lost cause to help them. However, there are some new tools and techniques, combined with a new awareness grounded in scientific insight and a lot of determination, that can help you to both support them in a healthy way and take care of your own needs. It all begins with understanding and compassion. The addict is quite simply someone who has lost their way in the world, usually because of traumatic events in their own lives, whether those are in the distant past or in their more recent history. Now, they're caught in a whirlwind of confusion. They might want to quit, but they feel helpless. It's a nightmare of epic proportions, but there is help.

No matter how long you've lived in the shadow of addiction, it's never too late to change. Your relationship doesn't have to fall apart while this happens, either. The light of love and compassion can guide you as you try to mend and rebuild your relationship. You can learn from these difficult challenges and restore your life to a hopeful and loving state. You might be able to do that with your partner or you might ultimately have to go your own way, but either way, you will grow your compassion, learn the blessing of forgiveness, and whether apart or together, you can give your partner the support they need as they move through the various states of addiction. Your true love and compassion can shine a light on the path that will lead them out of the darkness should they choose to follow it. If not, it will hold the space of acceptance, understanding, and profound compassion for them as they continue to struggle.

In this book, I will help you understand addiction from your partner's point of view. I will also explain the biology of addiction and how that can be a helpful tool for recovery. I'll discuss the connection between narcissism and addiction and the red flags of use and abuse that you need to look out for so you can take care of yourself, too. It's all too easy to forget that addiction causes trauma for you as well, and you must take steps to protect yourself if you are to have a prayer of helping your partner.

I'll also help you understand the foundations of true love and how to establish or reestablish them in your relationship, no matter how bad it is. I'll explain the things you should avoid doing as you try to help your loved one, as well as a better way to be helpful. I'll help you understand how you can take your power back and how to establish healthy boundaries that will protect you and your partner. It is a difficult journey to undertake. You will have to face many challenges, but where there is love, there is also hope.

I am living through this nightmare myself, and I understand where you are. I know the pain and disappointment you're feeling as you try to help your loved one overcome the monster that is addiction. But, there is a way forward, and it can lead to a happy, fulfilling life together. The journey to a better, brighter future begins here and now. Let's get started.

WHO IS ADDICTION

It's a burning need that won't be denied. It feels like a fever that is consuming my entire body. It's all I can think about. It's a constant craving that demands satisfaction. It promises relief if only you feed it, but it lies. The craving is never relieved; it is never satisfied. It drives my behavior. I feel like I would do anything to find that relief. I'll spend all of my money, I'll turn away from my family, and I'll steal--and maybe even worse--to get what I need. I do need it, in fact, as much as I need the air that I breathe. I used to enjoy the sensation, but now it's a terrible rash on my soul. I no longer like it, but I still want it, I need it. It's a nightmare from which there is no waking. I'm trapped in a web of lies--I even lie to myself--and constant need, constant craving.

This need has been in my life for so long now that I can't remember what it was like to be without it. There was a time before the need took over, but that was long ago, and I can't even remember how it started. It might have happened because I wanted to fit in with my peers at school. I didn't want to be the nerd who was afraid to try it. There might have been traumatic events in my early childhood that I don't want to have to confront, and to avoid that, I am running away from my own feelings. The demon that is addiction promised me I could hide in its warm embrace. But that warm embrace has become a torture chamber, and a need that can never be met.

Now, my days blend together in a constant search for relief. I am an empty vessel that yearns to be filled, but which can never be sated. I can't bring myself to face my family and friends, and so I don't think about them anymore. For me, their love and approval, if they were ever there in the first place, is nothing more than a distant memory. When they try to convince me to turn away from what I so desperately need, I stand firm in my conviction that they simply don't understand my pain. Truth be told, I no longer understand it, but I know I need it. I can't stand the thought of the disappointment my loved ones feel for me. I demonize them to quell my overwhelming feelings of guilt and shame. It has to be their fault I do this, because I can't face that it is my own fault. They must be making me do it with their constant nagging, their condescending attitudes, and their judgment. I will show them.

Somewhere deep inside me is a small, distant voice that tells me the truth. I just can't hear it clearly, and I find it hard to believe what it is saying when I do hear it. I shut it out because it confuses me. It is easier to detach from that small voice of sanity, because it wants me to do things I don't believe I can do. It wants me to face the demon, to fight it, and to free myself, but that seems too hard. The need is so strong; the voice of the demon is too sweet. I don't have the strength to resist. I am desperate to free myself, but everywhere I turn, the craving is my constant companion. Sometimes I wonder how I can even go on living, sometimes I think I shouldn't, and sometimes, when it is darkest, I think about ending it all.

Something is there though, inside me, something that keeps me from ending the pain. It calls to me. It wants me to know that I am more than an insistent craving, a constant need for external relief. It beckons me to look inward, to find my true self. Yet, it is just a lightened area in the dark sky of my addiction, like what you see in the sky in the hours before dawn. It isn't even a pinprick of light, but it's there. That gives me hope. Maybe there is a way out of this prison. But each time I dare to think of hope, the demon beckons, the need becomes ever more insistent, and each time--like the coward that I believe myself to be--I relent. I walk willingly back into that dark embrace. I gladly drink the poisonous nectar to kill the shame, to numb the pain.

Does any of this sound familiar? This is who addiction is. It's your loving husband, your beautiful wife, your precious child, your grieving father. You might never have talked to your addicted loved one about their point of view before. That's understandable. If you're not an addict, it's really hard to understand why they just can't quit. I know, because I live with an addict in my life, and I've wondered that very same thing. Like you, I didn't know how strong the grip of addiction really is, and I guess I never thought it would happen to someone I love, because it never happened to me. However, addiction can strike anyone of any age. Maybe your older spouse went into the hospital for an operation and came out addicted to painkillers. Maybe tragedy struck, and the grief caused them to use substances to numb the pain. How did addiction enter your life?

There are many ways addiction can become a problem. It has many names--maybe it even goes by your name or the name of your loved one. It has many faces. They used to be the innocent faces of hope and the potential of a bright future. That was before the demon addiction stole their promise. The sad fact is they are not alone in their plight. Almost 21 million Americans suffer from addiction. It steals their lives, it takes away their livelihoods, it eats away at their relationships, and it leaves them feeling isolated, worthless, and utterly rejected. Their pain isn't contained within them either; it spills out to any loved ones who dare to stay with them in their world. If that's you, the spouse of an addict, you know how it affects your life and your relationship. But what is addiction and why is it so powerful?

WHAT IS ADDICTION?

WHEN PEOPLE SAY that addiction is a disease, they are absolutely correct. In fact, it is a form of a brain disorder that results in an uncontrollable craving for a substance of some kind that will give the addict instant gratification. The strength of the craving is such that any consequences of engaging in the addictive behavior doesn't even register in the addict's mind. The addict is a slave to their drug of choice (which includes alcohol), but they frequently will switch to another drug if that is not available. Addiction can also involve activities like eating, sex, gambling, or working. Regardless of whether the addict is hooked on drugs or an activity, it is something that they cannot stop doing. That's what defines addiction. Is there someone in your life who meets this definition?

What's more, addiction is a chronic and life-threatening disease that cuts the addict off from family, friends, social engagements, and virtually anything else in their life. Addiction has a physical effect on the brain; it changes the way the brain responds to signals. It affects the chemical messengers in the brain (called neurotransmitters) in such a way that it causes the addict to be more fearful and feel pleasure more intensely, the latter of which tricks the brain into believing it needs the substance for survival. These changes can result in major psychological and physical effects including memory loss, paranoia, mood swings, confusion, weight loss, and poor personal hygiene. Additionally, addiction poses long-term health risks that can significantly shorten the addict's life.

HEALTH RISKS OF DRUG AND ALCOHOL ABUSE

The health effects of drug and alcohol abuse can be catastrophic. Aside from changing the brain's chemistry, substances spread throughout various body systems where they can cause permanent damage. The most common problems include the following:

- **Immune System Problems**: Various drugs, such as cocaine and alcohol, can negatively affect the immune system which makes the addict more susceptible to infections like HIV, hepatitis B and C, or any variety of bacterial infections. For example, approximately half of all patients with pneumonia have abused alcohol in the past, and those abusing alcohol have more serious complications and a higher rate of mortality than those who have not abused alcohol. Moreover, the euphoria associated with intoxicating substances like alcohol lowers inhibitions which increase risky behaviors like unprotected sex, which increases the likelihood of contracting a sexually transmitted disease.

- **Cardiovascular Problems**: Stimulants increase the user's heart rate, whereas substances that depress the central nervous system slow it down, and that, in turn, affects blood pressure. Having consistently high or low blood pressure can increase the risk of blood clots and other circulatory problems, which can cause a higher risk for certain conditions. For example, alcoholics have an elevated risk of contracting pneumonia, tuberculosis, respiratory syncytial virus infection, and acute respiratory distress syndrome.

- **Gastrointestinal Problems**: Substances ingested orally can do serious damage to the digestive system. They can cause indigestion, nausea, vomiting, constipation, gastric reflux disease, damage to the esophagus, and problems with malnutrition. Alcohol specifically is associated with reflux esophagitis, increased risk of gastrointestinal cancer, pancreatitis, a rupture of the lower esophagus that results in internal bleeding, malabsorption, and nutritional deficiencies.

- **Respiratory Problems**: Any kind of drug that is smoked can damage the lungs and make them more susceptible to infections. Other drugs can cause shallow or irregular breathing, and a persistent lack of oxygen created by this breathing pattern can lead to organ damage. Alcohol abuse is associated with an increased risk for community-acquired pneumonia, such as that caused by *Streptococcus pneumoniae*.

- **Liver Damage**: The liver has several functions including nutrient metabolization and detoxification of substances that are consumed. Because drugs and alcohol are processed by the liver as part of the detoxification function, these substances can cause severe damage to this critical organ and lead to cirrhosis of the liver or hepatitis. Cirrhosis is also a risk factor for developing liver cancer.

- **Kidney Damage**: The kidneys also filter toxins from the bloodstream, and thus, they are affected by anything a person consumes. Drugs and alcohol can clog the filtration system or damage the tissues, which can overwhelm them and damage their ability to filter toxins effectively, a condition which will then cause a buildup of toxins in the blood.

- **Neurological Problems**: Consistent substance abuse leads to a brain disorder that results in changes to the areas of the brain associated with reward and pleasure, decision-making, and impulse control. Depressants, such as alcohol, reduce the excitatory brain signaling mechanisms which, if done long term, can lead to problems with movement, cognitive impairment, and memory loss. Stimulants like cocaine increase the firing of nerve cells that produce more physical energy and emotional highs, but once these drugs leave the body, the user crashes, often experiencing numerous negative side effects, and the brain will be slower at restoring the balance to neurotransmitters (those chemical messengers) like serotonin, dopamine, and norepinephrine. Imbalances in these chemical substances can lead to severe depression and other neurological disorders.

WHY DON'T THEY QUIT?

The simple answer is they can't, at least not without some help. If you're not an addict, it's hard to understand why someone would take the risk given the possible health effects and all the other negative consequences of their habit. For the addict, there is an overwhelming need for their substance of choice. They don't view it as making a choice between you and the substance they need so badly. They can't see it that way because the burning need to use their chosen substance clouds their reason. For that same reason, they also don't see the damage it's doing to you and other family members and friends in their life. It's quite simply an awful ordeal for everyone concerned. Are you caught in this vicious trap?

JOURNAL YOUR PAIN

Throughout this book, I want to give you outlets to express your feelings about your own situation. One thing that's helpful is writing in a journal. I know you might feel resistance to that, but before you roll your eyes, journaling has incredible power. It lets you fully express your feelings in a private and completely safe setting. You can say what you want without fear of anyone judging you in any way. You can pour out your pain onto the pages of that journal. I want to suggest you give it a try, because I believe you'll find it's a great way to help rid yourself of the pain that's been stored inside you throughout this hurtful situation.

As I said, I know how it goes. At first; you deny your loved one is an addict. You refuse to see what's happening. You make excuses for them; you tell yourself they're just having a difficult time right now, it's not an addiction. Once they get a job, or recover from that illness, or get over their grief, things will get better. But as time passes and that doesn't happen, you slowly start to realize it's not a passing stage. As you come to accept the truth, that your loved one is an addict, you then begin to strategize how you will convince them to quit. You practice the conversations in your head. You try to come up with the right words that will inspire them to quit. You think if you figure out the right thing to say, it will convince them of their own worth and they will make the decision to quit. You've heard that you can't make them quit, that they shouldn't quit for you, but for themselves, and that they will need to get help, but you think you and your loved one will be different. They can quit with your loving support without needing rehab or counseling or even a 12-step program. You're certain you can convince them.

You approach them in different ways. You threaten, you cajole, you bargain, you shame, and you give them ultimatums, only to fail to follow through. Nothing works. What's worse, you're caught in a trap, because despite everything that's happened, you still love them. A part of you hates yourself for being so weak. You may think, "Why can't I just leave them? Why don't I just walk away? Why don't I tell them to get out and never come back?" But you can't. You fear if you do, they will sink even deeper into their addiction until they lose themselves completely. You see yourself as the only thing between them and utter ruin, and you really still love them. All the while, the abuse (emotional and maybe even physical) keeps coming. You're being traumatized, and if you don't want to or can't bring yourself to get out of the situation, you need to express that pain as part of taking care of yourself. Journaling can help.

If any of this resonates with you, then trust me enough to try writing about what you're experiencing. It will help you to clear your own body and mind of the toxic effects of living with an addict. The truth is, the addict's manipulative logic can convince you that you are the crazy one, and you need to know you're not. Writing about what's happening can help you to see that. Just give it a try. Start by writing about the following topics:

- How the addiction got started;
- How long it has been going on;
- What the substance of choice is;
- How often your loved one uses;
- How it changes his or her behavior;
- How you feel when you know they are under the influence;
- Where you feel that in your own body;
- How it affects your own self-esteem.

This is the start of a long journey where you will have to confront some very difficult feelings, but you've taken the first step, and that's the most important one. It will get easier, you can heal, and only then do you stand a chance of helping your loved one.

CHAPTER SUMMARY

In this chapter, we've discussed the addict's point of view as well as the dangers of addiction. Specifically, we've covered the following topics:

- How the addict perceives their own addiction;
- What exactly addiction is;
- The health risks of addiction;
- Why the addict can't quit;

- How journaling can help you as you try to help
  your loved one.

In the next chapter you will learn about the biology of addiction, and how that might help as you try to find ways to help your loved one.

2

THE BIOLOGY OF ADDICTION AND HOW IT CAN HELP

Most people who are not addicts can't fathom the reason why, given the multiple negative consequences for addictive behavior, the addict wouldn't just simply quit. It's hard to understand when you see the addict literally risking their life for their habit. However, when you understand what is happening biologically when someone is addicted to drugs or alcohol, it becomes easier to understand why they can't just simply quit. It all starts in the brain.

THIS IS YOUR BRAIN ON DRUGS (OR ALCOHOL)

While that subheading is a play on a famous US public service announcement (that pictured eggs frying in a pan to represent what happens to the brain on drugs), the announcement is accurate insofar as the effects that addiction has on the brain. While biology is not the only factor in addiction, it is a major reason why people can't quit easily even when their habit becomes life-threatening. You might think that it's the substance that causes the problem, and while some substances are highly addictive, that fact is related to the changes those substances are causing in the brain. In essence, you're not addicted to the substance as much as you are to the chemicals that the substance causes your brain to release. Your brain is your body's supercomputer. It is a dynamic and complex organ, the proper functioning of which is critical for your survival. It helps us adapt to changing environments, and that quality is one important factor in the development of an addiction. Addiction fundamentally changes the brain in the following ways:

- It changes the brain's natural balance, something called homeostasis;
- It alters brain chemistry;
- It changes the normal communication patterns;
- It changes brain structures and their functioning.

It's helpful to examine these changes in-depth, to fully understand how much addiction changes your brain's functions. But first, let's discuss what the brain does to help us survive.

THE BRAIN'S NORMAL FUNCTION

The human brain has been evolving for millions of years. Humans have the largest brain relative to body size of any organism on the planet. As a species that is comparatively helpless--we don't have sharp teeth or claws, and we can't outrun our predators or our prey--our brain has made the difference in our survival. It is our superpower. In order to help us survive, the brain performs numerous critical functions. First, it is geared for problem-solving. It is constantly monitoring our environment looking for threats. When a threat is perceived, it induces physiological responses that prepare us for either fighting or fleeing. It ramps up your heart rate, speeds up your breathing, dilates your eyes, and shunts blood to necessary parts of the body so that you are able to either fight or flee. You may have heard incredible stories of someone performing a superhuman feat, like a mother lifting a car off of a child. Those feats are possible because your brain stimulates the release of certain chemicals or hormones like adrenaline.

The brain is also our storage system. It stores memories of various things that can help with survival. It remembers where food is located, and it also recalls good experiences versus bad experiences. It urges us to engage in good experiences repeatedly, and it helps us avoid repeating the bad ones. It also helps us focus our thinking by creating habit routines for the overwhelming majority of our daily tasks. For example, you probably don't think much about it as you brush your teeth. You no longer need to focus on how to move the toothbrush around your mouth. You engage in that activity more or less on autopilot. When you were first establishing that habit, you did focus on it, but once the habit was in place, your mind was free to think about other more important things. Much of your daily activity is habitual. You probably don't think much about driving to work, or taking a shower, or even starting your coffee maker in the morning. These are all habits that you do almost automatically. That's what defines them as habits.

HOW ADDICTION DAMAGES THE BRAIN

When addiction takes over, there are a number of ways in which the brain's proper function is affected.

1. **Addiction results in changes to the cerebral cortex**. The cerebral cortex is the area of the brain associated with higher thinking. These changes

impair decision-making and enhance both impulsivity and compulsivity. So while your decision-making skills are hindered, you are also more likely to do something impulsively, or without considering the consequences. Moreover, you experience urges to compulsively (as if you were being forced) engage repetitively in the behaviors associated with the addiction.

2. **Addiction alters the brain's reward system**. As our species was evolving, the brain's reward system was responsible for encouraging us to repeat pleasurable behaviors like eating and sex. That was good, of course, because it helped to ensure our survival as a species. But when this system is hijacked by addiction, the user experiences the drug or alcohol as pleasurable, and that engages specific areas of the brain that register pleasure, as well as other areas that stimulate desire or cravings. The latter is particularly important because even as people no longer experience pleasure from their habit, those areas of the brain that stimulate cravings can still be active. Thus, the addict can want their substance of choice even though they no longer like it. Those cravings are a major reason why it is so difficult to quit, and why so many people relapse even though they have the best of intentions to quit.

3. **Addiction is integrated in your memory and associated with good emotions**. The area of the brain called the amygdala is associated with memory and emotion. Your memories of an experience affect whether your brain will encourage you to repeat it or not. It's part of how your brain helps you establish habitual behavior. For example, let's say that you have a habit of coming home from work

and having a drink. Your brain stores this as a pleasant memory associated both with stopping work and starting to relax as well as with the pleasurable feeling you get from consuming the alcohol. After repeating this several times, finishing work and coming home become the cues for initiating the habit routine of having a drink. Those cues are powerful motivators to engage in the habit. If you try to stop, your brain registers the withdrawal as a negative memory and strongly encourages you to resume the habit. So here you have two factors that are encouraging you to keep engaging in the behavior: 1) the memory of the pleasant experience when using, and 2) the memory of the negative experience when trying to stop. That makes it very difficult to quit, and if you give in and relapse, the brain registers the relief experienced as another pleasurable memory, adding yet another source of encouragement for engaging in the behavior.

4. **Addiction damages the brain's ability to regulate stress**. The area of the brain that regulates stress is the hypothalamus. Most addicts use drugs or alcohol as a means of relieving stress, and if they try to stop using, it creates stress. That's a vicious cycle. You use to relieve stress, stopping creates stress, and using diminishes the brain's ability to regulate stress. Once again, that's a powerful motivator to continue using.

These effects on the brain help to explain why people with an addiction ultimately lose control over their actions. Their brain is screaming at them to continue to use their substance of choice. It began with a pleasurable memory recorded in their brain, then it became a habit, and stopping creates negative memories. All of which work together to encourage the user to continue. To illustrate how difficult this is for someone who's never had an addiction, imagine you are told you have to give up your very favorite food in all the world. If it's something you habitually eat, it makes quitting even harder, because your brain is hardwired to expect that pleasurable experience. To get what it wants, it will stimulate cravings that can literally fill your mind. It becomes all you can think about. If you've ever been on a diet, you have probably experienced this, and you most likely know just how difficult resisting those cravings can be.

It's a common misconception that the addict is choosing to use or that they are simply morally bankrupt around this issue, but as research has shown, the brain is actually changed as a result of addictive behavior, and the more you use, the more disruptive the problem becomes. The brain's normal, adaptive, and healthy behaviors of encouraging pleasurable activities and discouraging negative ones are hijacked by a substance that makes the brain perceive pleasure despite the health risks associated with the substance. Once hooked, those systems cause you to want more and more, and make you feel anxious when you're not using. By that point in time, the addict is using more to avoid the negative sensations than to experience the pleasurable ones. The more you repeat the behavior, the more damage is done to your decision-making center in the brain, which helps you ignore the harmful side effects. In fact, brain scans show that addicts have decreased activity in the prefrontal cortex where this decision-making takes place. That can cause them to use their substance of choice, even if the price of using is extremely high. But, of course, their continued use can cause severe damage to their body as well as the brain.

WHO IS LIKELY TO BECOME AN ADDICT?

Scientists don't yet fully understand the genetics involved with addiction. There is no one gene that causes or prevents addiction. There are most certainly genetic influences on addictive behavior, and we know that because addiction tends to run in families. In fact, The American Society of Addiction Medicine (ASAM) states that as much as 50 percent of the likelihood you will develop an addiction is determined by your genes. That is why the ASAM has defined addiction as a "chronic disease of the brain." However, not all members of an affected family will become addicts, as there are many other factors involved. As with any complex behavior, genetics can explain a part of it, but there are a number of environmental and personal factors that can play a role, too.

Being raised in a home with addicts, childhood abuse, exposure to extreme (often prolonged) stress are all factors that are known to contribute to alcoholism or drug abuse. Of course, the earlier you start engaging in these behaviors, the more likely you are to develop an addiction. Teens are particularly vulnerable given that their brains have not fully developed, particularly in the frontal region where impulse control and risk assessment take place. Additionally, the pleasure circuits in the adolescent brain are in overdrive, which makes the substance even more rewarding.

It's definitely a complex problem, one that requires dedicated, long-term treatment to beat. But there is hope because the very biology that helps create the addiction can also help beat it. Before we discuss that, though, let's examine the non-biological factors that impact addiction.

NON-BIOLOGICAL CONTRIBUTORS TO ADDICTION

As we've seen, the biology of addiction creates strong cravings for the substance of choice, which temporarily relieves the desire, but once it leaves the addict's system, negative emotions associated with withdrawal emerge and the brain begins creating strong cravings once again. In this way, the brain reinforces both the urge and the need for the substance and the behavior the addict engages in when using. To disengage from this habit, the addict will have to stop using and resist the cravings until the brain's neural patterns can reset. More about that below, but along with the biology of cravings and relief, there are the underlying non-biological mechanisms that may have helped initiate the behavior in the first place.

Non-biological factors that can contribute to drug and alcohol abuse are varied and equally complex. They include things like a history of child abuse, issues of self-esteem, medical problems, and even something as simple as needing to stay awake. Take the case of Adam. Adam was what you would call a Type A personality, a real go-getter. He was in school and running his own successful business at the same time. He never had problems with any kind of substance abuse, but his obligations began to pile up to the degree that they further exacerbated a mild attention-deficit problem he had. To combat his fatigue, he began taking stimulants to help him stay awake and clear-headed. That progressed until within two years of his first use of stimulants, he was smoking crystal meth several times per day. As you might imagine, this had devastating consequences. It disrupted his sleep patterns, he couldn't think straight, and his customary rational mind was replaced with fantastical whims. His business fell apart, he had to move in with his dealer, and his relationship with his daughter deteriorated. Ultimately, he needed a hit every hour or two to keep his high going. By that point, Adam was no longer enjoying the drug, but he still wanted it.

Aside from the biological feedback loop that makes it difficult to stop, there are other problems created by addiction. Social isolation gives the addict fewer people with whom they can connect for help or healthier pleasures. It's also not uncommon for addicts to rationalize that they're so bad or misunderstood that they should just continue their bad behavior. For example, Adam rationalized that all he had lost and his ongoing self-destruction was a punishment for his failures. It's not only the addicts that think like that; many people think of addicts as weak or morally corrupt. Their judgment reinforces the addict's own self-criticism, making it even harder for them to seek help.

The thing is that addiction is not about rational choices, moral character, strength, or the lack thereof. Addiction is, at its core, all about habit formation. While the addict does have to resolve underlying problems like issues with self-esteem or depression in order to be successful at recovery, they also have to break the habit. That's where the biology of habit formation can be useful.

HOW HABIT FORMATION CAN HELP TREAT ADDICTION

The formation of a habit is about repetitive behavior. There are three parts to habit formation. There is the cue (that's the trigger that initiates the habit routine), the habit routine itself, and the reward for engaging in the habit, which involves the release of brain chemicals like dopamine that create a pleasurable feeling. Earlier we used brushing your teeth as an example of a habit. When you were learning to brush your teeth, you began by doing it at certain times of the day; in the morning after eating breakfast, midday after lunch, and prior to going to bed. In those cases, breakfast, lunch, and bedtime are the cues or the triggers that initiate the habit routine. After eating breakfast and lunch, you experience an urge to brush your teeth, something you do with little thought now. The same is true as your normal bedtime approaches. In this case, it is the time of day that is the cue.

When you were initially learning the behavior and engaging in the behavior repetitively, there were changes going on in your brain. Each time you responded to the cue and performed the habit routine, your brain strengthened the neural pathways that ran the behavior program. It's like if you take a walk through the forest each day along the same path, that path will become more and more clearly established. The same thing happens with a habit. Those neural pathways, like the path in the forest, become clearer and easier for the brain's electrical signals to follow. As the brain establishes the behavior as a routine, special neurons take over to initiate the process and to end the habit routine when you're finished. Additionally, other neurons (called interneurons) act to prevent any other habit routine from running at the same time. They are active as you actually engage in the behavior. An entire system in your brain is dedicated to running this habit routine. It generates urges for you to engage in the behavior when it perceives the cue, it keeps your behavior focused on that single habit routine while it's running, and it terminates the routine when you're done. For most of our behaviors, this is a process that is helpful, but for addictive behaviors, this is the trap.

BREAKING THE HABIT

To break a habit routine, you have to do one of two things: 1) resist the urge to engage in the habit routine until the path becomes obscured through time, or 2) replace the bad habit routine with a good habit routine. The second choice will get faster, more successful results because you're using the body's same biology to assist you in creating healthier habits. With respect to addictive behaviors, as we've already mentioned, the addict has to break the habit routine while at the same time dealing with any underlying issues that initiated the habitual behavior in the first place. For example, Adam had to find a way to better manage his stress and mild attention-deficit disorder as well as break the habit routine of his meth use. Of course, dealing with underlying issues can require long-term psychological therapy, but you can still break the bad habit routine even if you haven't fully resolved the underlying issues. One great way this can be done is through habit stacking.

MAKING NEW HABITS

The key to replacing a bad habit routine with a good one is a step-by-step plan called habit stacking. This involves hijacking an existing habit routine and stacking a new routine on top of it, which allows you to use the already well-established neural pathways associated with your bad habit to begin stimulating your new good habit. Those same neural pathways will stimulate the good behavior just like they do the bad. This happens faster because your brain doesn't have to reinvent the wheel, so to speak. It won't have to clear a new path through the forest, it already has a path to follow-- the only thing that's changed is the habit routine itself.

For addictive behaviors, you might begin by stacking a new habit of waiting for 10 minutes on top of your old habit of substance abuse. The goal here is to eventually replace the bad habit of alcohol or substance abuse with a good habit that brings the same reward. Once you're accustomed to a short 10-minute delay before engaging in your bad habit, you can then extend the waiting period. Once you can successfully and repetitively wait that 10, 15, or 20 minutes, you can then stack a healthier habit on top of the bad habit. For example, if anxiety is the cue that triggers a desire for a drink, once you're accustomed to waiting for 10 minutes before consuming anything, you might add meditating during the waiting period. The meditation can help quell the anxiety just like the alcohol or drugs do, and eventually, you might be able to replace the bad habit altogether with the meditation.

Of course, this is a simplified example, but you get the idea. Over time, the urge to meditate would completely replace the urge to drink. Both behaviors yield the same reward in the brain, which is relief from anxiety and a shot of dopamine, the brain's feel-good chemical. Additionally, this happens much faster than creating a wholly new habit routine; in fact, it's possible to pick up the new habit in as little as 22 days, which is part of what makes habit stacking such a successful method for either creating new habits or replacing old ones.

WHAT IS YOUR ADDICT'S STORY?

This chapter has presented information about the biology of addiction as a way to help you understand why the addict in your life seems so helpless to stop their self-destructive behavior. But let's remember that it's also important to help you. It might be helpful for you to fully understand your loved one's problem by relating their story in your journal. What were the underlying factors that led to your loved one's addiction? Can you discern the cues that trigger their bad habit routine? Often, there is a time after finishing one routine where the pressure starts to build before they use again. What happens during that time? How does it affect you? How does this make you feel? Writing about your feelings can help you clarify the patterns and alleviate some of your stress.

YOUR HABIT ROUTINES

This is also a good time to look at your habit routines. It's quite likely that as your spouse cycles through their habit use, you also experience cues and habitual behavior as a result. Can you identify any habit routines--whether they are activities like sleeping, eating, or running away, or thoughts and emotions like depression, anxiety, or negative criticism of yourself or your loved ones? What can you do to replace bad habits with good ones? Perhaps stacking meditation on top of a sleeping or eating habit will help quell some of your building anxiety and fear. In your journal, identify one habit routine that you might begin to change, and create a step-by-step process for doing so.

CHAPTER SUMMARY

In this chapter, we've discussed the biology of addiction and how that can be used to help break habits. Specifically, we've discussed the following topics:

- The changes in the brain caused by addiction;
- The biology of habit formation;

- Some non-biological contributors to addictive behavior;
- How brain biology and habit formation can help break bad habits;
- Habit stacking to create new, healthier habits.

In the next chapter, you will learn about the red flags that indicate your loved one is using you.

3

FIVE RED FLAGS YOU'RE
BEING USED

LIVING with an addict is one of the most challenging relationships you can have. It's not at all uncommon for them to lie to you, emotionally abuse you, and sometimes even physically abuse you. Unfortunately, it's also not uncommon for them to steal from you. It may seem like they don't love you because they continually breach your trust, but it's important to remember that the addict doesn't think logically. It's not that they don't love you, it's that they can't express their feelings appropriately since their thoughts and emotions are all tangled up with the addiction. All they see is the need for a fix, and if that means they need your money or to lie to you, then that's what they will do. When you love an addict, you put yourself between them and their addiction. What can you do to best protect yourself? How do you know if you're being used? Before we get to that, though, let's do a little house cleaning.

DON'T BLAME THE VICTIM--THAT'S YOU!

The truth is there are more than five red flags that you're being used, but that could be a whole book on its own. Here we'll discuss the major red flags. It's not easy to accept that you might be unable to see how a loved one is using you. No one likes to feel like they're not able to pick up on when they are being used, but the truth is when you love someone, you want to believe they wouldn't do that to you.

One important thing to overcome is the idea that somehow you're a fool because you were lied to and you didn't realize it. Why would that make you a fool? Why doesn't our culture view the liar as a fool instead of the person to whom they told a lie? The truth is you're not a mind reader, and you can't always detect if someone is lying to you or telling the truth. Intuition can sometimes help and you should trust your gut instincts. However, it's not your responsibility to know when someone is lying to you. It's their responsibility to tell the truth.

So, let me say as forcefully as I can: it is NOT your fault if someone lies to you or uses you! It is NOT your fault for wanting to believe someone you love. Everyone deserves to believe in their loved ones, particularly those with whom we are most intimate. When you share your bed, your body, your love, your dreams, and your soul with someone, when you journey through life with them, you deserve to believe they are on your side. You deserve to believe they can be trusted. You deserve to have your partner walking through life's challenges with you. It's important to get that straight right off the bat. Now, let's take a look at those major red flags.

WHAT IS MEANT BY BEING USED?

When you think about being used, you probably think first about someone using you for money. While it is true that a loved one might use you for your money, being used means much more than that. It can also refer to being used for your enabling of their behavior, or for your labor taking care of your home and children. It's common for the spouses of addicts to bear the lion's share of the workload around the home. That might mean earning wages to pay the bills, but it can also mean doing the majority of the household chores, being the sole caretaker of the children, and/or being the only one in your relationship who engages in caretaking. We'll discuss enabling behavior in subsequent chapters, but suffice it to say that many addicts look for someone who will validate their addictive habits, who will, in essence, give them permission to continue engaging in substance abuse. They want someone to take care of them, but they often do not return the favor. These are all ways in which you can be used. That's not okay, and it's not something you should continue to accept, even if you are adamant about staying with your addicted spouse. If you feel that any of this applies to your situation, it's likely you're being used. That doesn't mean the relationship is beyond help, but if you choose to stay, you need to be fully aware of the red flags.

RED FLAGS

The red flags we'll discuss can be grouped into several main categories. In each category, there may be a number of behaviors to look out for. The categories are:

1. Moods
2. Stories

3. Schedules
4. Needs
5. Manipulation

It's important to examine each of these areas in more detail so that you can recognize the variety of behaviors you might encounter.

Moods

When someone is using you, one of the things you'll notice is the dramatic mood swings. They may be nice or loving one minute and stone cold the next. Their mood swings effectively keep you guessing, and pretty soon, you find yourself always walking on eggshells. These are games your partner is playing. Games are an ego default, particularly when having real feelings gets too scary. When the addict feels threatened, their ego kicks in, and they start playing games as a defensive maneuver. Authenticity can often be too difficult for the addict given that it requires inner confidence and a strong sense of self-worth, something many addicts lack. They know they're being manipulative, and they know it's hurting their relationship with you. This is what makes their inner world a pretty scary place full of self-judgment and fear of loss, and the feelings associated with all of that can swing wildly from displays of love and desire to flaring tempers. This means their inner world can make your outer world a pretty scary place, too.

It's important to remember that your partner is driven by constant cravings. Much of how he or she responds to you isn't truly personal. They're consumed by the need they have for their preferred substance. For example, they may start a fight with you so that they will have an excuse to leave the house and use. In this case, it's not about something you did, it's about getting their fix. Often, you might feel as though you're totally caught off guard. You might be having a normal conversation, for example, but suddenly, they twist it to find a way to blame you for something. The discussion escalates quickly into an argument, and before you know it, you're left feeling as if you are somehow to blame. It's a clever trick called gaslighting, a technique the addict uses to start an argument and manipulate your behavior. It's all designed to get them out of the house where they can use without any impediment, and it's helpful for their cause if they can keep you off balance. If you want to talk about something, they become an expert at diverting your attention to another topic. They know exactly which buttons to push to get you focused on something completely different, and it happens fast. It is something you have to be very consciously aware of in order to keep from following them down one rabbit hole after another.

Once you've recognized the games your partner plays, you will be able to control the automatic responses that his or her behavior instigates in you. That's a big step in the right direction. If you stop giving him or her the reaction they're looking for, you remove one of the many ways in which they manipulate your behavior. The best way to get a handle on those automatic responses is to remember this isn't about you or anything you've done--the argument is a ruse. Have compassion for your spouse, but stand firm when you see these kinds of erratic, emotional displays. You have a right to demand better treatment.

Stories

Another game that addicts play well is the sad story or "woe is me" game. They frequently engage in telling you just how hard they've had it as a way to garner sympathy. This feeds into other behaviors as well. They'll use the sad story to get you to do favors for them or give them money. The stories have a pattern to them, one in which the addict is always the victim. He or she didn't do anything wrong, they were simply the victim of circumstance or someone else's bad behavior. If you don't buy into their story and give them what they want, they often follow up with the cold shoulder.

It's important that you not believe their stories. If they don't get what they want frequently enough, they will eventually move on to another tactic. Still, it can be difficult to resist the temptation, because the stories are often quite sad. They seem so compelling, and because this is someone you love, you want to be on their side. You have to remember that even if something seemingly unfair happened to them, it is quite likely a case of self-sabotage. Addicts typically have a fear of achieving success in anything other than consuming what they're craving. They often will do something that they know deep down will sabotage that success. If you do yield to their demands and give them what they want, you're just helping them to continue using and engaging in their self-destructive behavior. This is called enabling behavior, and it's something that can be very difficult to stop, but it's critical that you try. We'll discuss this more in subsequent chapters.

Schedules

If your partner is using you, the only schedule that matters is theirs, and you'll likely find they spend an inordinate amount of time away from you. They won't care if you have plans or have something to do. They will have all the time in the world to spend with their friends, often while excluding you because their friends don't want them to quit their addiction. They may even see you as judging them. In reality, that's only because they're judging themselves. They may only spend time with you when it's convenient for them, and that doesn't happen very often, because they constantly want to use, and they see you as the judgmental stick in the mud that keeps them from doing that. If you do manage to plan something together, they often fail to follow through on those plans. This makes it almost impossible to plan anything. Everything you try to do with them is tainted by their need to soothe the demon inside of them.

Needs

Your addicted partner is unable to respond effectively to your needs. It doesn't really matter what those needs are--space, a desire to spend more time together, help with chores, or anything else--the addict won't be able to prioritize anything above their own needs. The truth is their addicted state makes them unable to focus on almost any task without a huge effort on their part. It's part of why you may feel they don't love you, but it really isn't that; they just can't express that love in a healthy way. Still, this can cause many serious problems in your relationship.

Manipulation

One of the addict's fortes is manipulation. Most addicts excel at storytelling for the purpose of manipulation. They might lie to get you to give them money, they might feign illness to get out of work, and they might even use mistakes you make against you at every turn. If you dare to defy them, be prepared for not just a cold shoulder, but an icy arctic freeze. They consistently hold you to a double standard. They will fail to complete their chores around the house, but be prepared for a huge fight if you bring it up. It could seem they are tired, ill, or angry every time you need or want something, but should you make the same claim, they aren't interested in hearing about it. Their emotional overreaction is the manipulative part of their game. If someone starts yelling at you every time you ask them to do a chore around the house, naturally, you're going to stop asking. That's manipulation. If you give in to any demand every time your spouse cuddles you and tells you they love you, they can use that behavior to manipulate you as well. With an addicted spouse, you have to be on the alert to how they are acting and the behaviors their actions are provoking from you. If you see a pattern, that is a good indication you're being used.

WHAT CAN YOU DO?

In the following chapters, we will discuss very specific actions you can take to care for yourself, but the purpose here is to help you understand what you're up against. You can't help yourself if you don't know the strength of the force that's driving the behavior of your loved one. It's as if they are under a spell, one that only allows them to see one, continuous, incessant, nagging craving that can never be satisfied. You can't change their behavior in the least. There is no threat, no inspiring words, no action or agreement you can make that will affect their desire, their need for that substance. That is their burden and their choice. Your burden is, in some ways, worse.

You must endure their pain and yours, too. They are unaware of the damage they do to you, but you feel it all the same, and you see their horrific struggle as well. You have to bear the burden as you attempt to support them through the healing process. Moreover, the scars will remain long after they are free from their addiction. It's not an easy path, and it's not even one you have to go down. You can choose to leave, and no one would blame you. If, however, you choose to stay, then you must practice good, continuous, healthy self-care. You have to understand everything you can about the addict's condition. The chapters to come will help explain more about addiction and take you through specific self-care steps you will need to take to retain some level of happiness and sanity as you go through this process with your addicted partner.

JOURNAL ACTIVITY

This is another opportunity to write in your journal and express your feelings about the red flags you see in your own relationship. Take time to express what you see happening. It will help you document the behavior, which will help you recognize and respond to the behavior appropriately. It will also give you the opportunity to let your feelings flow through you so that you don't follow them into the abyss. Write about the red flags you see. How do they manifest in your relationship? How does it make you feel when your partner engages in these behaviors? Are there steps you can take to set a boundary or express your needs to your partner in a way that won't bring an angry response? Writing about all of this can help you purge your frustration, document the patterns you see, and strategize appropriate solutions.

CHAPTER SUMMARY

In this chapter, we've discussed how you can tell if your partner is using you. Specifically, we've covered the following topics:

- Understanding what is meant by being used;
- Resisting the urge to blame yourself;
- The five red flag categories of behavior that signify you're being used;
- The importance of having all the pertinent information for making the decision on whether to stay or go.

In the next chapter, you will learn about how narcissism and addiction are intertwined.

4

NARCISSISM AND ADDICTION--
UNTANGLING THE MESS

MANY PEOPLE DON'T KNOW that there is a strong link between narcissism and addiction, but the two frequently co-occur. It can be very difficult to know if someone you love is suffering from both alcoholism and narcissism. Many behaviors are common to both problems. How can you tell whether your addicted spouse is also a narcissist? The first step is to understand what narcissism is and how it is tied to addiction.

NARCISSISTIC PERSONALITY DISORDER (NPD)

NPD is a mental health condition that causes people to have an unrealistic view of themselves. This unrealistic self-image is accompanied by a lack of empathy. The disorder causes symptoms that are emotional and largely social. The narcissist may be extremely arrogant and have an obsessive need for admiration, but this is typically masking a deep-seated sense of insecurity. Narcissists also have a disregard for social consequences and strong feelings of superiority, behaviors that are often shared with the active addict. Here are a few other typical characteristics of the narcissist:

- Manipulative behaviors
- Attention-seeking behaviors, especially in medical environments
- A demanding attitude
- Poor self-esteem
- Constantly comparing themselves with others
- Focused on obtaining special treatment
- An inability to get along well with others
- A deep need to be right
- An extreme need for admiration
- Impulsive decision-making
- Resistance to treatment

In addition to these behaviors, narcissists frequently demean other people to make themselves look better. They behave in ways that serve to elevate themselves with little regard for how their actions affect other people. They also tend to be very sensitive, and when they feel as if they have been wronged, they will become hyper-focused on the situation or the person who may have hurt or insulted them. The narcissist will also indulge in elaborate fantasies about how great they are, their past achievements, or their dreams for the future. Once again, these are often a cover for their low self-esteem.

Part of the problem with narcissism, however, is that despite the fact that the narcissist feels superior, they also tend to feel like outcasts. This is typical because of their antisocial behaviors, deep-seated feelings of unworthiness, and profound self-doubt, and those feelings and behaviors are part of why many people with NPD also struggle with substance abuse.

When two mental health conditions occur together, it is referred to as a dual diagnosis. What's more, the two conditions can also interact and influence one another. Narcissistic behaviors that are the result of deep-seated insecurities can influence the individual to abuse substances to mask those insecurities, and the influence of those substances can exacerbate narcissistic behaviors and feelings of insecurity. Given this negative feedback loop, it's not surprising that more than 40 percent of people diagnosed with NPD also have a substance abuse problem. Moreover, 30 percent also have a mood disorder, and one-third have problems with anxiety. Furthermore, people with NPD report high levels of shame, anger, and helplessness, despite the fact that they seem to be so arrogant. These problems probably stem in part from the fact that it's difficult for people with NPD to form meaningful and lasting relationships, and that's because the behaviors associated with narcissism are so destructive. It's a vicious cycle and one that becomes even more extreme when mixed with a substance abuse problem.

It's likely that many people who suffer from NPD get a sense of relaxation, comfort, and belonging when they abuse substances. The "high" also helps them mask the inner turmoil they're constantly experiencing. The inner turmoil is evident when you consider the dangers that people who suffer from a dual diagnosis face. They are at higher risk for suicide, domestic violence, criminal convictions, financial problems, a history of interpersonal violence, being sent to prison, and developing cardiovascular and gastrointestinal problems.

WHAT CAUSES A DUAL DIAGNOSIS OF SUBSTANCE ABUSE AND NPD?

NPD affects more men than women, but the exact cause is not clear. Genetics and neurobiology (the way the brain and the body interact) play a role, but there are also various personal factors that increase a person's chance of developing a dual diagnosis. An unpredictable home environment coupled with childhood abuse or neglect, traumatic events, early exposure to alcohol or drugs, other mental health conditions, extreme praise or criticism in childhood, unrealistically high expectations at home, or too much or too little attention from a parent or other authority figure are all situations that can increase an individual's risk for both narcissism and substance abuse.

WHAT IS THE TREATMENT FOR PEOPLE WITH A DUAL DIAGNOSIS?

It's very difficult to recover from either narcissism or substance abuse without help, but it's even harder to recover from a dual diagnosis. Treating either disorder without treating the other will make it almost impossible for the person to experience lasting recovery. Part of the problem is that standard treatment programs for substance abuse require people to admit their powerlessness over their addiction, but narcissists have difficulty admitting any kind of helplessness, and they certainly don't want to submit to a higher power. They may even think they are a higher power, and therefore, they tend to think they can handle it alone. That makes it very unlikely that they will succeed in a standard treatment program.

There are treatment plans for people suffering from a dual

diagnosis that provide a customized treatment plan designed to treat the whole person. These holistic programs allow the sufferer an opportunity to address each problem individually. Treatment often involves a combination of behavioral therapy with medications, and the research supports that this combined treatment is the most effective type of treatment for co-occurring disorders. It's also helpful for people to have several introductory sessions so they can get to know their therapist and to take healing at a slow, respectful pace. Through several conversations, contradictions in the patient's behavior become apparent. For example, when the narcissist says everything's under control, the therapist can gently point out the speeding tickets and arrests that have occurred in the recent past. In this way, the narcissist's denial can be broken apart, something that can help make it easier to maintain sobriety.

HOW DOES THE DUAL DIAGNOSIS AFFECT FAMILY MEMBERS?

For the spouse of a person with a dual diagnosis, it's a particularly difficult situation. A narcissist expects you to make them the center of attention, and substance abuse only exacerbates those demands. The underlying insecurity that plagues the narcissist is also a hallmark of a substance abuser. What's more, attempts to burst the narcissist's bubble of superiority are met with extreme defensiveness and anger. That's true whenever someone tries to give them a reality check, and of course, the addict is equally averse to a reality check.

It's not uncommon for the spouse of a narcissist, like the alcoholic's partner, to learn to tread lightly. They often ignore inaccurate statements and lies, go along with their fantasies of greatness, and stroke their egos with compliments and praise. It requires constant work on the part of both the narcissist and the people in their life to maintain their elaborate fantasies. To that end, the narcissist prefers the company of people they can manipulate, both physically and mentally. They want people around them who will provide them with the constant validation they need, someone who will confirm their superior status without fail.

Since they lack empathy, they feel no sense of wrongdoing when they manipulate or outright abuse others. Because they believe themselves to always be right, they believe this gives them the license to treat others in any way they see fit. They only see life from their own perspective, and thus, if there is some disagreement, they are confident they are right. They simply don't understand why someone would be upset with them. If someone asks them to change, they believe that person is just being selfish or perhaps, they are jealous of the narcissist's superior abilities. It's emotionally dangerous for them to acknowledge any wrongdoing or need to change. They believe everything that goes wrong in their lives is due to someone else's wrongdoing. If they had to admit fault, that would create an intense, painful inner conflict. That means the spouse often bears the brunt of the blame in the relationship.

In short, loved ones of a narcissist are expected to provide unconditional support, constant praise, and to comply with each one of the narcissist's desires. As the spouse of a narcissist, you will be expected to go along with their version of reality. If you fail to meet those demanding needs, the narcissist will view it as betrayal and respond accordingly. Adding substance abuse to this type of personality disorder is like touching a lit match to gasoline, and the results can be explosive.

This is a very difficult situation to live with, especially since it really requires professional help to resolve. The spouse of a partner afflicted with either condition is likely to be seen as the root of their problems, and when the two problems are combined, it will be very hard for a spouse to make a transformational impression on the addict. Even leaving them is seen as the ultimate betrayal, something to which they respond with anger and resentment. The best thing that the spouse of a sufferer of both conditions can do is help that individual seek professional help. There is a frightened, insecure, even child-like person hiding somewhere inside the dual diagnosis prison, but helping them into the light of love, self-confidence, and self-worth requires the delicate touch of an objective, experienced therapist.

If a spouse simply continues to bend to the will of the narcissist addict, it is very unlikely they will resolve either problem. To continue to give in to their demands in order to keep the peace, while understandable, is simply enabling their bad behaviors. You aren't helping them, and you certainly aren't helping yourself. It's a hard truth to accept when you love someone and when you know the real person hidden behind the mask, but by accepting your own helplessness in the face of their narcissistic addiction, you stand a far better chance of helping them find the light in recovery.

JOURNAL ACTIVITY

Do you think it's possible your addicted partner is also a narcissist? What kinds of behaviors suggest that might be a possibility? How is it affecting your family? What solutions might improve the situation? Let yourself write freely about the behaviors you're seeing. Include in your writing communication strategies for talking to your partner about the problems you see. You don't have to follow through on these, but by writing about what you would like to do, it can help to express that anger and your fears, and that can help develop real solutions.

CHAPTER SUMMARY

In this chapter, we've discussed the common link between narcissism and substance abuse. Specifically, we've talked about the following topics:

- Narcissistic personality disorder (NPD). What it is and the typical characteristics of those who suffer from this condition;
- The dual diagnosis of NPD and substance abuse;
- What causes these problems;
- What the treatment is for a dual diagnosis of NPD and substance abuse;
- How a dual diagnosis affects family members, particularly spouses.

In the next chapter, you will learn how to establish and maintain a foundation of true love with an addicted partner.

5

THE FOUNDATION OF TRUE LOVE
WITH AN ADDICTED PARTNER

LAYING the foundation for true love is hard even when both partners are healthy, but it's even more challenging when your partner is an addict. Still, the basics are the same as they are with any other relationship. If you can establish a strong foundation, it will help you maintain your love connection even through the worst of times. The following foundational rules will help you to keep your love alive.

- **Unconditional acceptance**: This is one of the most difficult things to do in any relationship. What this means is accepting the person you love as they are, *not as you want them to be*. This doesn't mean accepting inappropriate behavior, but it means understanding that no one is perfect. It also means getting that fairy tale idea of Prince Charming or Cinderella out of your head. You have to accept your spouse for the person they are, warts and all. For the spouse of an addict, that means accepting their addiction, and understanding that there is nothing you can do about it. That's one of the most difficult parts of unconditional acceptance, accepting that you can't change your partner. You want to help, but the reality is you have to accept them as they are, and support them to make better choices. This might be too difficult to do, and if it is, it might be time to consider leaving. If you choose to stay, however, you have to accept who your partner is unconditionally.

- **Respect**: Respect means considering the wishes and needs of others. It means understanding what your partner needs and not judging them for their preferences. Once again, this is difficult to do when your partner wants and needs something that is not healthy for them. Again, your instinct is to help them, but they have to confront the reasons for their own self-destructive tendencies if they're ever going to change. You should support that, but you can't force it.

- **Honesty and trust**: These are the bedrock of a healthy relationship. To generate trust, honesty is a must. This is something that almost every addict has trouble with because they often lie out of shame for their behavior. They are tortured by their reliance on their substance of choice. They understand it's destroying them and you, and it's that knowledge that brings them such pain and shame. So they lie. That will undoubtedly compromise your trust in your partner.

Perhaps the best way to handle this is to refrain from judgment. That doesn't mean you accept being lied to, but it does mean you show your partner that you understand why they engage in this behavior. For yourself, you have to practice acceptance that this is how your partner is with their addiction. You have to look beneath the pain and shame the addiction is causing and see what's really there--the divine and loving person trapped by their own insatiable need.

- **Communication**: It's difficult to have good communication without honesty, but if you can practice non-judgmental communication, you might get your partner to open up and face some of their issues. If they can begin the process of understanding the reasons behind their addiction, this will be the first step toward healing. The most important thing you can do is keep the lines of communication open. You want your addicted partner to know they can talk to you at any time, no matter the topic. Let them know you will be there to listen to their pain without judgment and without trying to convince them to do something they aren't ready to do. It can also help to model good communication by opening up to them about some of your fears and issues. When they see that you trust them, it will make it easier for them to develop trust for you. With trust as a foundation for communication, you can open up to each other, and that can do wonderful things for your relationship.
- **Compromise**: This is another necessary element for a happy relationship, but it can be difficult for the addict. There is no compromising with the demon, but this is something that you will need in order to continue trying to save your relationship. You'll have to decide how much you're willing to give on a particular topic and then discuss with your partner having him or her meet you halfway on that. It might help if you come to the negotiating table after

having already thought about what you ideally want, what you will accept, and what is an absolute deal-breaker.

- **Consistency**: This is one area that will greatly assist your addicted partner. Threats to leave him or her or vacillating between love and hate will exacerbate your spouse's desire to use. Remember that beneath that addicted outer shell, beneath the narcissist's bravado, there lives a frightened, vulnerable person. Any threat to their equilibrium is a seemingly catastrophic possibility. They don't react rationally, because the substance blinds them to logic. Unfortunately, you'll have to be the one who responds with love, calm, and consistency. If you show them that, while you won't enable their bad behavior, you will be there to support them, and that will go a long way toward helping them stay calm. When you know what to consistently expect from one another, that allows each of you to open up and express your true feelings. That is the road to healing.

- **Work together**: Let your partner know you're on his or her team, you love and support them, and you want to work with them toward the goal of a healthy, happy relationship. It's also important to be willing to pick up the slack if your partner falters and expect the same from them. Help them focus on the goal with you and keep moving toward the realization of that goal.

- **Listen**: Listening can be even more important than speaking. Active listening techniques involve listening to your partner as if everything they say is true and repeating back what you hear to ensure you have a full understanding. Try to listen to what your partner is really saying to you without becoming defensive or judgmental. Listening is one of the greatest skills you can develop for any relationship, but it's doubly important for a relationship that involves an addict.

- **No comparisons**: Mark Twain said, "Comparison is the death of joy," and truer, wiser words have never been expressed. There will always be someone in a better position, someone prettier, someone richer, someone healthier, and so on. You'll never win the comparison game, and for an addict, constantly comparing them with someone else is a strong trigger for use. They will simply think, "Well, if I'm so bad, I might as well get drunk or use drugs." Comparison is a death knell for any relationship, but it's more tragic for one that includes an addict because it strikes at the heart of their low self-esteem issues. Instead of comparing yourselves with someone else, create your own relationship goals, and work toward those. Don't look outside your relationship for markers, use your own milestones to measure your success.

- **Affection and compliments**: If you lose the affection you once had in your relationship, you have lost the relationship. Everyone needs to feel loved and loveable. It's even more critical to show your affection to your addicted partner. Despite their disease, there are many things you still love about them or you wouldn't be staying with them. Tell them about it and let them tell you why they love you. Love multiplies love, so be generous with your compliments and affection. Show it often to remind yourself about all the reasons why you fell in love in the first place.

- **Speak each other's love language**: People give and receive love differently and understanding what your partner considers evidence of love is vital to the health of your relationship. Some people feel loved with a lot of physical contact while others feel you're showing your love if you frequently give them little gifts. Still, others need compliments to feel loved while some people need you to do something they can't do to show you love. There are many ways people show their love, and it's important to know what both you and your partner consider evidence of love.

- **Grow together**: You might have an addicted partner, but that doesn't mean that you can't grow together as you strive to meet your relationship goals. Part of the goal will be to have a healthy, happy relationship, and that can be very difficult for the addict to achieve, but if your partner is at least trying and moving in the right direction, that's growth. It may be a small amount of growth, but as long as you're going forward rather than backward, you're heading in the right direction. It's helpful for achieving growth to leave the past in the past. Don't bring up past wrongs in your relationship, but rather stay focused on the present moment.

RULES FOR FIGHTING FAIR, EVEN WITH AN ADDICT

As we've already mentioned, addicts are experts at manipulation and deflection. That's not because they're malicious, it's because they're addicted. That's why it's a good idea to establish a few rules of engagement to make sure you can stay focused on the current problem and work toward a solution. Everyone in every relationship fights from time to time, but there is a way to fight fair rather than following a scorched earth policy. These will help you express your feelings without hurting your partner. It's always tricky with an addict because they're extremely sensitive, but if you can get them to agree to the following rules, it will help you both learn to fight fair:

- **Apologize when you're wrong**: If you're wrong, own it. It doesn't make you vulnerable, it makes you strong. Put yourself in your partner's shoes. By doing so, you will set a great example for your partner to follow, and you'll maintain your own integrity.
- **Forgive easily**: This is where empathy can really be helpful. By understanding what they're going through, when they apologize, you'll find it much easier to forgive them. Remember that everyone is human, and we all make mistakes, which will make it easier to forgive any wrongs.
- **Being right is not the most important thing**: Love is more important than being right. Sometimes, the better part of valor is to let go of the need to be right, and instead show your partner that you love them. Choose your battles carefully and check your ego at the door. That may be hard for the addicted partner, but here is where you can set an example that lets them know you're in it for the long haul.
- **No name-calling**: If a fight descends to the level of name-calling, it's time to step back, take a break, and come back to discuss the issue when things have calmed down. Relationship experts refer to criticism, defensiveness, contempt, and stonewalling as the four horsemen of the apocalypse. When these show up, they are

extraordinarily destructive, and if you're engaging in these tactics commonly, it's far more likely your relationship will end in divorce. Even a five-minute break can be enough to reset your temper and help you return to the conversation in a more positive frame of mind. This is a particularly important rule if you're in a relationship with an addict. Their ego is very fragile and name-calling is very damaging. It's also damaging to you, so if your partner starts calling you names, it's time to walk away.

- **Don't generalize**: Avoid using phrases like, "You always do that..." Those kinds of phrases disempower the current conversation. You want to stay focused on the matter at hand. Referring to past arguments or behavior raises your partner's defenses and shuts down the lines of communication. It's a common distraction technique for the addict, meaning it will be your responsibility to ignore it when your addicted partner brings up something from the past. You'll need to insist, instead, on staying focused on the present moment.

- **Use "I" statements**: Don't say, "You make me feel…," instead say, "I feel…" The reality is that your partner doesn't make you do or feel anything. You are responsible for your own feelings and actions, so when you're expressing yourself, say things like, "I feel worried when you are late. I think something might have happened," or "I feel angry when you accuse me of being unfaithful." These arouse less defensiveness in your partner, and they also remind you that you have the power to change your reactions. This is a way for you to take ownership of your own feelings and improve your communication with your partner.

- **Fighting is not failure**: It's hard to live with someone else, no matter who they are, and it's even more difficult when that person is an addict. Conflict is a natural part of relationships. No one is perfect and something will always come up. By setting the rules of engagement for fighting, you can express your disagreements in a respectful, loving manner. This is someone you love and they presumably love you too, so being respectful and loving even when you disagree should come naturally.

HOW TO SET RELATIONSHIP RULES

To set clearly defined relationship rules, you'll want to examine your own emotional landscape and actively practice self-awareness as you determine what you feel is the right way to disagree. Your partner should do the same. You want to avoid reactions to provocations and knowing what triggers your partner helps to prevent that. Take responsibility for yourself and insist your partner does the same. Both of you will feel better for having done so, and your fights will probably be more respectful and productive as a result.

Remember that to be respected, you first need to respect yourself, so follow through on what you say regarding disagreements. For example, if you say you'll walk away the first time they call you a name, then follow through on that. This will also help you prevent yourself from projecting your own fears onto your partner. Setting up relationship rules won't stop your fighting, but it will help you disagree in a far more respectful and healthy way. This is one of the most important building blocks for moving forward in your relationship.

JOURNAL ACTIVITY

For this activity, begin by writing about what it was that attracted you to your spouse in the first place. Where did you meet? What was the first thing you noticed about him or her? When and where was your first kiss? When did you know you were in love? What is your partner's love language? What makes them feel loved? What makes you feel loved? Is it the same or different than your partner? Do you express your love for your partner in a way that will make them feel loved? Do they do the same for you?

Now, write about when your problems started. When did you first realize your partner had a problem with addiction? What kind of denial behaviors did you use in the beginning? How is the addiction affecting your true love relationship? How is it affecting other members of your family? Are you still able to grow together? What might you do to get back to that foundation of true love you started with? Write out some things you could do to set new relationship rules and reestablish your foundation of love. Be specific and come up with at least three strategies you can implement in the next week. Don't forget to express your feelings for each part of this activity. Be honest with yourself about the state of your relationship.

CHAPTER SUMMARY

This chapter has focused on building a strong foundation for true love, even with an addicted partner. Specifically, we've discussed the following topics:

- The foundational rules for true love;
- How to fight fair;
- Setting strong, clearly defined relationship rules.

In the next chapter, you will learn what not to do in your relationship with your addicted spouse.

6

DON'T DO THAT, DO THIS

IT IS EXTREMELY FRUSTRATING to live with someone who is consumed by their cravings, and whose singular focus means your needs will largely be ignored and you will often be the one to blame for any problems. You may end up feeling hurt, angry, and confused. It feels overwhelming, but there is hope. Recovery is possible, and there are ways you can help your loved one to heal. How do you do that? You're already walking on eggshells, which makes it difficult to approach your loved one. While there are no set guidelines on helping someone overcome addiction, there are some dos and don'ts. The following guidelines can help you as you approach this delicate subject.

DON'T LOOK DOWN ON THEM

It's understanding to be upset with your loved one as you watch them consumed by their addiction, but you need to understand that addiction is a disease. You wouldn't judge someone for having a different kind of disease like cancer, and you shouldn't judge them for their disease of addiction, either. There is already enough stigma around addiction, and the last thing the addict needs is those closest to them looking down on them for something they don't feel they can control. Avoid blaming them for their addiction; instead, practice acceptance and empathy.

DON'T BLAME YOURSELF FOR YOUR SPOUSE'S ADDICTION

It's not uncommon for your spouse to try to blame you for their drug or alcohol use. They might say things like, "You make me mad and that makes me drink," or "Now I'm going to drink because you started an argument." It's important that you realize this is denial and distraction at work. Their problem is just that, their problem. There is nothing you have done that has caused their addiction. They have to take responsibility for their own actions, and you also need to acknowledge it is their responsibility. Let go of feeling as though you have control over the situation. They control their own actions, and both of you have to realize that.

DON'T IGNORE THE PROBLEM

It can be hard to accept that someone you love is afflicted with an addiction. You'll likely be tempted to ignore the signs of addiction or explain them away. It's easy to make excuses for their behavior, but this is not going to work. You're not helping them if you try to reason that they're just going through a tough time or that they'll "snap out of it." If you're going to have any hope of helping your addicted loved one to recover, you have to face the problem head-on, don't ignore it. Addiction is a progressive disease, the addict will only get worse over time--the more they use or drink, the worse the problem becomes.

DON'T TRY TO FORCE THEM TO QUIT

Tough love rarely works when it comes to addiction. Giving your spouse an ultimatum might work for a little while, but until they are ready to get sober, they are likely to return to using as soon as they can. The addict has to quit because they want to quit. That's the only way they will be able to achieve a long-lasting recovery. If you force them into recovery, it is unlikely to last, and they will come out of it feeling resentment towards you.

DON'T DRINK OR USE DRUGS WITH THEM

It might be tempting to just give up and go along with them, but this will only exacerbate their problem. It won't solve the addiction, and it will have a negative impact on your health, something you can't afford with everything you're already doing. You'll also want to keep your own mind clear while interacting with your addicted spouse.

DON'T COMPROMISE YOUR WELL-BEING BECAUSE OF YOUR SPOUSE'S ADDICTION

If your spouse becomes violent with you while they're under the influence, get out, and get help. You should never compromise your physical well-being. It's also important to take care of your mental well-being. Your addicted spouse will try to make you think you're the one with the problem. Don't buy into that kind of distraction. Make sure you have someone you can talk to about this problem so that you have an outlet for your emotions.

DON'T GIVE UP

By now, you might be thinking that things sound pretty glum, but there is hope, so don't give up. The last thing your addicted spouse needs is to hear that you don't believe they can beat their addiction. If you give up on them, they will probably give up on themselves as well. It's hard to fight an addiction, but it's not impossible. Your addicted loved one will need support as they try to do this. Your support can make all the difference in the world.

DO EDUCATE YOURSELF ABOUT ADDICTION

If you haven't had to deal with an addiction problem in the past, you might want to educate yourself more about it. The more you know, the more you can help your addicted spouse. There's also support for family members of addicts. Check out the websites for the National Institute on Alcohol Abuse and Alcoholism (NIAAA), the National Institute on Drug Abuse (NIDA), and the Substance Abuse and Mental Health Services Administration (SAMHSA). These are excellent resources that can give you information on getting help for both yourself and your loved one.

DO ADDRESS THE ISSUE

You are going to need to have that difficult conversation with your loved one. Confronting them about their addiction can be intimidating. To prepare for this conversation, it's a good idea to speak to a professional. They can give you tips on how to best approach the addict. Additionally, it's best to broach the subject when they are sober since trying to bring it up when they're high or drunk will only result in anger and frustration for both you and your spouse. It's also helpful to write down everything you want to say. As we've discussed, it's common that the addict will use distraction to get you off track when talking about this problem. If you have something written down, it will be easier for you to keep the conversation focused. Finally, try to remain calm, be open and honest, and let them know you love them and want them to get better. Tell them that is why you're having this conversation--because you care.

DO SEEK COUPLES COUNSELING

When you're dealing with an addicted spouse, it's more than just your feelings that get hurt. With each angry interaction, your relationship is damaged. Your loved one might not be willing to seek treatment for their addiction, but they may be willing to try couples counseling. Couples counseling can help to open up the lines of communication between you and your spouse, and it can help you express your feelings of frustration with the situation.

UNDERSTANDING CODEPENDENCY

Another very important concept you need to understand is codependency. Some people struggling with an addicted loved one, particularly spouses, end up in a codependent relationship. Codependency happens when you desire to show love and help your addicted spouse, but that help can end up furthering the addiction. In the long run, this can be very damaging. How do you know if you've become codependent?

There are a number of signs to look out for. Here are several red flags:

1. You take responsibility for the addict.

People who are codependent frequently feel that they are responsible for the decisions, actions, and even the thoughts of their partner. They want them to feel happy, even at the expense of their own happiness. They often feel a need to protect them. For example, they might drive them to and from the bar so they won't get a DUI, or they might call their boss for them when they are too hungover to get to work. They will also make excuses for them, all to keep them out of trouble. The codependent spouse typically does all of this at their own expense. Does this apply to you? Be honest with yourself about how your own actions might be enabling your partner's addiction.

2. You put your addicted spouse's feelings first.

Codependent spouses put their partner's feelings before their own. They will frequently ignore their own feelings or beliefs in order to accommodate their loved one. This often manifests as self-neglect. That only makes the situation worse. Is this something you're doing? Are you ignoring your own values or beliefs so that your addicted spouse will be happy or stay calm?

3. You stay in the relationship out of fear of abandonment.

Codependent spouses often fear abandonment. They're afraid of being alone and rejected. They also often desperately seek approval, and to get that, they constantly try to please their addicted spouse. The fear of abandonment is so strong they may even give their addicted spouse money, drugs, or alcohol just to keep them around. Are you afraid to be alone? Do you ever appease your addicted spouse so you won't be alone?

4. You have trouble talking about your feelings.

A codependent spouse becomes so accustomed to burying their own feelings as they seek to appease their addicted loved one that it becomes difficult to even recognize their own feelings. They have a very difficult time expressing any feelings of fear or dissatisfaction, and they also have difficulty talking about their own needs and how to meet them. They're focused solely on "fixing" their loved one rather than getting the help they need. Can you express your feelings freely? If you find yourself struggling to express your dissatisfaction or anger, this applies to you.

5. You're unable to set personal boundaries.

Codependent people are unable to say no to any request their partner makes, even if they're not comfortable with what the request is. They want to believe that puts them in charge of the situation, but the reality is they are only helping the addict achieve their goal to use. Are you able to set boundaries? Do you follow through on enforcing the boundaries you set?

Even if you weren't codependent when the relationship began, it's easy to become codependent as your spouse struggles with drug or alcohol addiction. Breaking the iron grip of codependency means seeking treatment.

TREATING CODEPENDENCY

It might seem difficult to tell the difference between true love and codependency, but when you're attending to the needs of another without consideration for your own, it's a sign of codependency. If any of the above signs apply to you, you'll want to think about if you're in a codependent relationship, and if you are, you'll want to know what treatment options are available.

Codependency is a learned behavior. You might have learned it from watching a codependent parent or through the experience of living with an addicted spouse or loved one. Often it's a combination of the two. Children who grow up with a parent who is codependent or with parents who are both emotionally unavailable are at higher risk of being codependent. They seek out relationships similar to what they have seen modeled by their parents. They seek out an emotionally unavailable partner, something typical of addicts, and then they stay in the relationship because they believe they can change the person. In a sense, they are trying to "fix" the relationship they had with their parents, which, of course, is something they can't do.

The subconscious hope of the codependent person is that their spouse will see the love they are giving them and be inspired to change. They believe that if they can just hang in there with that person long enough, their spouse will give them the love they wanted from their parents. The reality is that can never happen. The time has passed, and that kind of thinking is destructive because the codependent partner doesn't have healthy boundaries to protect them from the physical and emotional harm that an addicted spouse inflicts. Even more problematic is the fact that the codependent spouse may not even realize what's happening. They never learned what true love looks like, so they continue to live in a loveless relationship, hoping for the best.

It sounds like a hopeless situation, but it's not. If you have identified with the codependent red flags listed above, you can heal from codependency. To have a loving, healthy relationship, you must do just that. The good news is that because codependency is a learned behavior, which means it can be unlearned. If you really want to keep the relationship, you will need to heal yourself from any codependency first. Here are a few healthy steps you can take to help yourself heal:

- **Start with honesty**: First and foremost, be honest in your communication with your partner. If you don't want to do something, say so, and if you don't mean something, don't say it. Just like your addicted spouse is responsible for his or her behavior, you are responsible for yours too. So take responsibility by being honest with yourself and your spouse.
- **It's not personal**: Most codependent people take everything very personally. You have to remember that your addicted spouse is responding to the constant craving they feel. You need to accept that reality, and part of doing that is understanding it's not personal.
- **Take a break**: It's okay to take a break from your partner. It's healthy to have your own friendships, and you should take time to spend with your friends. Doing so will help you express your feelings, and it will remind you of who you really are. It's also helpful to spend time with other family members. They're usually a good support network,

and along with your friends, someone you can turn to when things get difficult.

- **Consider counseling**: If you can get into counseling with your partner, that would be best, but even if not, you can seek out counseling for codependency. Such programs will give you the support to set better boundaries and take better care of yourself. It's always helpful when you can see that other people are struggling with some of the same problems. Just like there are alcoholics anonymous or narcotics anonymous support groups, there is a codependents anonymous support system to help people heal from codependency.

JOURNAL ACTIVITY

For this activity, write about whether or not you're codependent. Do you make excuses for your spouse and enable his or her behavior? In what ways do you do that? Do you take responsibility for their actions? Are you afraid they will embarrass you in front of your friends? Do you feel they will look down on you for that? Do you have an inner critic? What kinds of things does that Negative Nellie say to you? Take this time to write down some of the ways you treat yourself badly. Now, strategize how you can improve your situation. What don'ts have you done? Write them out and then write out a statement where you recognize your humanity and forgive yourself for handling the situation in an inappropriate way. Acknowledge that this is a tough situation for anyone to be in, and you're doing the best you can. Be kind to yourself--don't let any negative sentiments enter into acknowledging your humanity.

CHAPTER SUMMARY

In this chapter, we've discussed tips for what to do and not do in a relationship with an addict. Specifically, we've discussed the following topics:

- The kinds of things you shouldn't do when in a relationship with an addict;
- The kinds of things you should do when in a relationship with an addict;
- What codependency is;
- How to know if you're codependent;
- Steps for treating codependency.

In the next chapter, you will learn about setting boundaries and regaining your power in your relationship.

7

BOUNDARIES AND POWER IN YOUR RELATIONSHIP

IN THIS CHAPTER, we'll delve into the topic of boundaries in order to discuss how to determine what boundaries you need to set and how to set them. When you have trouble setting boundaries, it's also often true that a power imbalance has developed within the relationship. For that reason, we'll also discuss how you can regain your power. Let's begin with boundaries, what they are, how to set them, and which ones to set.

Addiction involves numerous fear-based behavior patterns and dysfunctional interactions within the family. There's everything from the need to control others, perfectionism, hanging on to resentments, or behaving like a martyr. There's anger, disappointment, frustration, and sadness. Setting boundaries can help to improve familial interactions and communications. That's a first step toward healing some of the damage caused by the addiction. Many people wonder, however, what exactly is a boundary?

WHAT IS A BOUNDARY?

A boundary is quite simply a limit that people set in order to protect their overall well-being. It can be a physical or emotional boundary, and setting healthy boundaries helps people define who they are and what they require in a relationship to feel safe, supported, and respected. Unhealthy boundaries can also be put into place. These are behaviors or thoughts designed to manipulate or control people. A simple statement from family dynamics trainer, Rokelle Lerner, helps put the concept of healthy boundaries into perspective: "What I value, I will protect, but what you value, I will respect." That's the essence of healthy boundaries.

WHY ARE BOUNDARIES IMPORTANT?

Boundaries express our personal needs and values, and they give us space to express ourselves as individuals as well as what's most important to us. They provide a set of guidelines for communication with others; they let people know what behaviors are acceptable and unacceptable to us. Boundaries can be very difficult to set and maintain when addiction enters the picture, but they are arguably never more important. As the spouse of an addict who might be codependent, you might wonder if boundaries can work in that setting. The answer is yes, even in a codependent relationship, boundaries can work to identify where you end and the other person begins. As a codependent spouse, you can use boundaries to identify your needs, which can help you to take care of yourself.

It's important to understand that you're only setting boundaries for yourself. The other people in the relationship will also get to set their boundaries in accordance with their needs and values. By identifying your needs as you set your boundaries, it makes it easier to understand both your needs and your partner's needs, and if your addicted partner is trying to set unhealthy boundaries that represent an effort to manipulate or control your behavior. Thus, even in codependent relationships, setting boundaries is a vital part of creating healthier interactions.

WHAT ABOUT BOUNDARIES AND TOXIC RELATIONSHIPS?

Toxic relationships are defined as those that involve behaviors that cause physical and/or emotional harm to one another, and as you can imagine, they are very common in relationships involving addicts. These types of relationships typically involve intense shame, dishonesty, severe manipulation, and physical and/or emotional abuse. If you're in a toxic relationship, it's likely there is a general disregard for one another's values and needs. It's also typical that boundary violations run rampant. Still, it is in these relationships that it is even more critical to establish healthy boundaries to ensure your safety and continued wellness.

WHAT ARE SOME EXAMPLES OF SETTING HEALTHY BOUNDARIES?

There are some situations where it is evident that boundaries are immediately required, such as in those relationships where violence or other types of abuse are present. These are obviously in need of strong boundaries, but there are also numerous situations where boundary violations might be subtle. You might, for example, justify your spouse's inappropriate behavior or blame yourself for their drug or alcohol use. These are cases where you are not respecting your own boundaries. With so many ways in which boundaries can be violated, it's a good question to ask how you can recognize a situation that might require a stronger boundary.

Check in with yourself and try to recognize any discomfort you're feeling in your body as well as notice what kinds of thoughts you're having. Here are a few things to look for:

- Is your stomach in a knot? That's your body telling you the situation is uncomfortable and not good for you.
- Do you feel angry or resentful? If you find yourself feeling this way, that can indicate you might be asking too much of yourself. You need to say no in a kind way.
- Do you feel confused? Perhaps you're feeling manipulated, which could indicate you need to take some time to more carefully consider your involvement in the situation.

Our values guide us in which boundaries to set, and that's where you should look to decide on your needs. For example, one good boundary to set with a loved one is to refuse to lie for them. If lying goes against your values and it makes you feel bad about yourself, it's something you shouldn't do. If someone asks you to lie for them, you need to consider your values and how doing what they're asking would make you feel. If it's something that causes discomfort for you, either physical or emotional, then it's a place where a boundary needs to be set. You need to refuse that request.

Another area where it might be good to set a boundary is around your own use of alcohol or drugs. While you are not an addict, you should consider whether drinking an occasional glass of wine with dinner is more important than helping a loved one in recovery. If your relationship is more important, it's a good boundary to set to refrain from using yourself when your addicted spouse is around. If your own use is more important, then it might be helpful to reconsider whether you should stay in the relationship and/or whether you might have a problem as well.

For your addicted spouse, he or she will need to consider how important sobriety is for them. They need to strategize how to protect their own sobriety if they're in recovery, particularly when they are likely to encounter situations where other people will be drinking or using drugs. They will need to plan for how and when to leave in order to prevent a relapse.

HOW TO SET BOUNDARIES

The first step to setting a boundary is to ask yourself what the motive is for setting that particular boundary. This could be a very difficult question because you might have lost touch with your own feelings, needs, and well-being. You might have some difficulty distinguishing between setting a boundary because it is consistent with your needs and values and setting a boundary because you think it is better for the needs of your addicted spouse. You want the motive to be about self-care rather than a desire to control or change your partner. If you feel confident this is the case, you're ready to set some healthy boundaries.

The next step is to communicate the boundaries you want to set, and this can be tricky given that many addicts react with anger when someone sets a boundary. This is particularly true if you've been enabling their behavior up to this point. One of the best pieces of advice is simply to say what you mean and mean what you say, but don't say it in a mean way.

Words and manner matter when you're trying to communicate your boundaries. Be honest, but respectful, and try not to be confrontational. By communicating your boundaries in that way, it's more likely your addicted spouse will listen to what you're saying.

As you're communicating your needs, remember to use "I" statements; rather than saying, "You make me...," say, "I feel... when you..." Using these kinds of statements is less likely to provoke a defensive response, but the end goal of setting a boundary is to make sure the person understands that you are not okay with their behavior. Toward that end, you also need to clearly state the boundary. For example, "I feel frightened when you drink and drive. Because I am frightened, you may not drive my car anymore, and I need to tell you that I will not bail you out if you get arrested for driving while under the influence." With this kind of statement, you're taking ownership of your feelings and you're clearly stating the boundary you're setting.

Just because you use "I" statements doesn't mean your partner won't react with anger, frustration, or denial, but as long as you're coming from a place of genuine self-care, you'll be better able to respond to their reaction without trying to fix it. In this example, you've expressed your feelings, you've stated the boundaries you're setting, and if your spouse reacts with anger, you can simply explain that you will not be a party to their self-destruction because you love them. Again, it's a statement of your own feelings rather than trying to fix their reaction or their feelings about your boundary.

WHAT BOUNDARIES SHOULD YOU SET?

There is no one-size-fits-all with boundaries because every situation is unique, but there are some general boundaries that can help ensure you and your children live in a safe environment, even when it includes an addict. The following boundaries will help establish a safe space for you and your children:

- **No drugs or alcohol around me, the children, or in the house**: It's important to let your spouse know what is and is not acceptable in the home. You have to communicate that clearly so you can feel safe and secure in your own home. You should also clearly state the consequences if your spouse violates the boundary. Will you force them to go someplace else? Will you call the police? Will you call other family and friends to help you enforce the boundary? Make sure your spouse knows what will happen in the event they choose to violate the boundary you've set.

- **No alcoholic or drug-using friends allowed in the home**: The addict's friends are often a trigger for your spouse's use, and you don't want one addict in the house, let alone more. Setting a boundary that keeps his or her substance-abusing friends out of the home will help reduce the damaging effects of addiction.

- **I will not bail you out or pay for a lawyer to defend you**: This puts the responsibility for the consequences of their actions solely on the addict. It is the addict's responsibility to help themselves. By setting this kind of boundary, you are communicating to him or her that they are an adult and will need to take responsibility for themselves.

- **No insults or ridicule**: By setting this boundary you are communicating that you are no longer willing to sacrifice your self-worth in this relationship. This will help to reestablish your self-respect and integrity and establish a standard of treatment from others. You have the right to expect decent, respectful treatment.

- **I will not give you any more money**: This is you communicating that your money will go toward the things you value. You can use it to pay the bills you need to keep a roof over your head and the lights on, but it puts the responsibility for paying their own bills on them, which means he or she will have less money for their substance of choice. This doesn't mean they will quit using--and you shouldn't be setting the boundary for that reason--but it does mean that you won't be paying for their use anymore. You're protecting your physical well-being and your finances with this boundary.

- **I will not lie or cover for you under any circumstances**: We've discussed previously, but it's important to remember that the disease of addiction thrives on chaos and lies, and setting this boundary will help remove you from the mayhem. Your loved one will have to take ownership of their own behaviors and make their own excuses or face the consequences of their actions.

- **If you're not on time for dinner, you're not welcome to join us**: It's not uncommon for spouses of an addict to hold dinner until they finally show up or even end up making two dinners because of their tardiness. That's an example of you putting yourself last. If you allow this to happen, you're allowing the addiction to take over the lives of your family. Take back what's important to you. If you're responsible for dinner, then let your spouse know when it's served, and if they're not there, let them get their own dinner.

Setting boundaries is critical both for you and your loved one. It's easy for the chaos created by addiction to take over your life, and that can cause you to lose track of your own well-being. By setting strong, clear boundaries, you can get off the emotional roller coaster and reclaim your sanity, your healthy life, your self-respect, and your stability. By setting a healthy example, you'll also give your addicted spouse more reasons to seek help. You will have to hold firm to your words and promised actions. You don't want to make idle threats or your addicted spouse will take advantage of that in the future.

One problem that can crop up as you attempt to set boundaries is that the balance of power might be off in your relationship. Romantic relationships are complex and dynamic, and the power balance can be tricky. There are differing power roles in every relationship, but if the two of you lose sight of those roles, you might find you're giving up your personal power. It's essential to restore the balance of power to find your way back to a healthy relationship.

To take back your power, you have to take responsibility for your own happiness. Part of doing this means setting those boundaries as we've discussed, but it also means that you no longer settle for less than you deserve, and you stop allowing your partner to have the upper hand. You become the author of your own story once again, and in doing so, you reclaim your own happiness.

POWER ROLES

Relationships are defined by dynamic power roles that shift with the changing seasons of your partnerships. These roles can be defined by many things, and it is up to each partner in the relationship to determine specifically what works for them. When there is a problem with that understanding, it can lead to an imbalance of power, and that can make it hard to thrive as a couple. If you allow an outside party to control or manipulate how you think, act, or feel, you are giving up your power, which will ultimately lead to unhappiness all around.

If your relationship is unbalanced, it's not happy, and it won't survive long term. It's important for both parties in a relationship to strive for maintaining equilibrium while also encouraging each other to get their own needs met. Clearly, introducing an addiction into the relationship can easily throw this balance of power out of whack. If you have given up your power, however, it's not too late to get it back. You can take charge of your own life again and reclaim your power within the relationship.

HOW DO YOU LOSE POWER?

Losing power in a relationship with an addict is a process; it doesn't happen all at once. Often, the wild mood swings and chaos in the relationship conditions you to behave and think in certain ways to avoid rocking the boat. There may also be elements of your past relationships or childhood experiences that factor into your power loss as well. Once you understand how you're behaving, you can begin to make a plan to get your power back. Here's a look at some of the characteristics that come into play with losing power:

Low Self-worth

Low self-worth is something that often happens to the spouse of an addict. You get used to putting yourself last and placing a lower value on what's important to you. Moreover, you come to believe there is no value or merit in your own authenticity, you don't trust your decisions, and you feel unable to strike out on your own or to even take responsibility for your own happiness or unhappiness. As you lose confidence in yourself, you can easily miss a power shift occurring in your relationship. You have to learn to trust and love yourself in order to be able to accept the reality of your own situation.

Societal Pressure

Society puts a lot of pressure on any couple to conform to a set of cultural expectations for relationships. This pressure is much stronger than you think, and when the relationship includes an addict, you may feel pressure to keep up appearances based on society's view of a good relationship. You might feel pressured to hide your spouse's behavior or make excuses. You feel as though you have failed if other people find out your spouse is an addict. That's not, after all, the ideal societal picture of what a relationship should be. This creates an imbalance as the addict rarely cares about societal pressures, but they are certainly willing to let you work hard at keeping up appearances. Society may also believe that certain roles should exist in your relationship, based on gender or status or some other factor. When you feel pressured to be part of an unbalanced relationship, you can find yourself engaging in the behaviors that will create exactly that kind of relationship.

Abuse

A partner who bullies or belittles you can also simply take your power away. These kinds of behaviors are not uncommon in the addict, and thus, there is often a dramatic power shift as a result. You perpetuate this unbalanced relationship when you accept that kind of treatment. This is where boundaries are critical for stopping the abuse.

History of Trauma in your Relationships

If you have had traumatic relationships in the past, or if your parents modeled a traumatic relationship for you, then you might have learned that equal partnerships don't exist and that you shouldn't ask for what you want. Essentially, you've taken on a skewed view of what love should look like, and that can cause you to attract abusive partners or accept it if your addicted partner takes your power away.

WHAT DOES A LOSS OF POWER LOOK LIKE?

A lack of power can look very different depending on your specific relationship. You might let your partner make all the decisions or they might bully you. A few of the typical indicators that you've lost your power include the following:

- **You never call the shots**: If you never get to make decisions, regardless of the situation, that indicates you've given up your power. When one person is in control of all the major and minor decisions in your life, you're no longer taking personal responsibility for your decisions and your opportunities. If this is true for you, you're no longer dealing in your own personal power. That can put you in a very dangerous situation.

- **Externally defined moods**: If your moods depend on the moods of your loved one, that indicates you relinquished your personal power in the relationship. Your own happiness should come from within, and it shouldn't be dependent on anyone other than yourself. It's easy for an addicted spouse to manipulate your moods and cause confusion and conflict. In that kind of environment, you can lose your power quickly without even realizing it's happening.

- **Always giving in**: If you are always the one who gives in to what your partner wants, you have most likely sacrificed your power. You're allowing your partner to have more "space" in the relationship. Since an addict already occupies a large amount of relationship space, you can't afford to lose anymore.

- **Fluctuating self-worth**: Do you find that you're feeling great about yourself one day and terrible the next? That can indicate you're relying on external sources for personal validation. If you truly value yourself, that doesn't change even with changing external circumstances. An addicted spouse can cause a fluctuation in your self-worth, and they will certainly take advantage of it to get what they want. You have to find your own validation from within to reclaim your power.

- **Unable to set boundaries**: We've talked about boundaries and how to set them in this chapter, but if you find you're unable to do that, it could indicate you've given up your power in the relationship. Moreover, if you can't stick to your boundaries, your addicted spouse will probably take advantage of that to take away your power.

- **Constantly redefining yourself**: If you're always changing your self-definition based on what other people want, it's another sign that you're looking for external validation. Other people's definition of happiness may not fit your definition of happiness. You must take responsibility for your own life and your own happiness. If you're always changing to fit in with someone else's definition of what life should be like, you'll always go down the wrong road. You have to look within and discover your own definitions regarding life satisfaction.

- **Settling for less**: Settling for less is, in some ways, the very definition of giving up your personal power. You're sacrificing what you truly want, perhaps out of fear that you'll never get what you truly want, so you better take what you can get. By doing this, however, you're giving up your chance at independent happiness.

- **Unable to speak up**: If you don't feel like you can speak your mind, it's likely because you feel like you don't have the power to do so or you don't think it's safe. To be truly happy, you have to be able to speak your truth. Expressing your feelings truthfully is the only way to build a stable, equitable, and lasting relationship. An addicted spouse will often try to keep you from doing this because they don't want to hear the truth about themselves. They can even actively try to suppress your ability to do this, which means you'll have to insist on speaking up frequently.

- **Needing to ask permission**: It's always true that when you enter a relationship, your choices should be made after considering how they will affect your partner. That's part of being a team, but that doesn't mean that your partner has the right to tell you what to do. If you find that you have given up the right to make your own decisions to your partner, then you've given up your power. An addicted partner may try to take your power through pressure or intimidation, which means you will have to establish very strong boundaries.

WHAT ARE THE CONSEQUENCES OF GIVING UP TOO MUCH POWER?

When you give up your power in any relationship, there are many consequences that range from losing yourself to losing your relationship. It's important to understand this concept so that you can fully understand why it's so important to reestablish your power. One of the most obvious consequences is that you lose yourself. You find you don't know who you are or what you want from life anymore. This causes identity obstacles, disillusionment, disappointment, and resentment. Moreover, the longer you allow yourself to be ruled by someone else, the worse the situation gets. You will start to feel as if you're intolerable to yourself and your self-worth will suffer. You have to know yourself to truly love yourself, and you have to love yourself to love others.

It's also true that unbalanced relationships where one partner dominates rarely stand the test of time. They tend to be more superficial and even parasitic in nature with one partner draining the life and happiness out of the other. Without mutual cooperation and respect, the appearances soon break down and contempt comes to rule the relationship. All of this is more profound when the relationship involves an addict. This also leads to resentment over the missed opportunities for love, shared experiences, and joy. You'll come to find your life intolerable, and you'll soon find yourself looking for an out. If you think about yourself in 30, 40, or 50 years looking back on your life, what do you want to have accomplished in life? How would you feel if you find that you're looking back at a sea of other people's accomplishments and dreams? Will this make you feel as if you've lived the life you came here to live? When you give up your power, you give up the adventure of living your own life. So, what can you do if you find you're giving up your power?

HOW TO RECLAIM YOUR POWER

There are a number of things you can do to reclaim the power you may have given up. Of course, one of the first ones--and I know it sounds like a broken record--is to set and maintain strong boundaries. These are the ways you express your values, your beliefs, and your desires for your life. You have to fight for those boundaries, and by that, I mean wage war for them. These are what define you; they show the world what you value and that you value yourself. Follow the advice above and state your boundaries in clear, honest terms, and back them up by following through on stated consequences. To truly establish good boundaries, you'll need to do a few other things to take back your power.

Another thing that helps you reclaim your power is to become the author of your own story. Don't let anyone else, not even your spouse, call the shots in your life. You'll have to step out into the unknown because now you'll be taking full responsibility for your life. You'll be responsible for defining what you want and getting it. You'll have to let go of external validation and rely on your internal self-worth and guidance. If this is new to you, you can start small by choosing three things each day that you will do entirely on your own. It's also helpful to get out on your own, even if that means taking a short walk or a bubble bath in the other room. Get by yourself and become comfortable being by yourself. The more comfortable you get with being on your own, the more comfortable you will become calling your own shots. You'll also find you have incredible internal strength and that will help you realize that you're the only one who should be validating your joy, your life choices, and your definition of success. As you grow stronger in your self-reliance, you can take charge of your own life and story, you can stop letting your partner write your story. That may mean you stop reacting to your addicted partner's mood swings or bullying tactics, or it may eventually mean you decide to strike out on your own. Whatever it means, make it your story with your own happy ending.

To take control of your own life, you'll need to increase your self-confidence. When you have low self-confidence (meaning you don't believe you can do things successfully) you end up with low self-esteem, or a low opinion of your-self. Low self-esteem damages the way you see your role in your relationship, and that also affects the way your partner sees you, too. You have to find your own personal strength to boost your self-confidence and self-esteem. To boost your self-confidence, start celebrating small things you do well each day. Congratulate yourself and take note of how well you were able to do the small tasks--maybe it's making dinner or doing the laundry, but it's an accomplishment that you completed successfully. By acknowledging that you've successfully completed these small tasks, you'll build your self-confidence to the point where you'll be ready to take on larger, more difficult tasks.

Another part of building self-confidence lies in not allowing others to tear you down. That includes you. Celebrate your strengths and accept your weaknesses, but look for the lessons they offer. It also helps to realize that everyone is human with their own set of strengths and weaknesses. You're no different, and just like everyone else, you deserve love, self-respect, and to be treated kindly. Sometimes, to do this, you have to confront some pain you suffered in your past. You have to face it, accept it, and let it move through your body so you're no longer trapped by it.

The next time you find yourself feeling frightened or anxious, stop and turn around as if you're seeing yourself in the corner. Approach yourself with kindness and ask yourself, as if speaking to a child, "Why are you frightened (or anxious or angry or whatever the emotion)?" You'll be surprised at what comes to you. When you get the answer, give yourself the reassuring kindness you should have received when the past trauma happened that made you so fearful. Begin with understanding by telling yourself, "I completely understand why you would feel that way. That was a frightening event in your life, but you don't have to be afraid anymore. I'm here with you now, and together, we're stronger than ever before." This might sound simplistic, but it really works. You're essentially giving yourself the love you should have received when the trauma originally occurred. This will help you recover your self-worth, stop defining yourself by the terms of others, and understand that you are good enough just as you are.

Once you're able to see your real worth, it's often much easier to stop wasting time on other people's dreams. You'll start pursuing your own dreams which will help you reclaim your power and increase your life satisfaction. You only have a short time on this planet, and you don't want to waste the time you have going after something someone else wants you to pursue. You might choose to spend it in service of others, but that will only be successful if you can establish strong boundaries, value yourself, and if it is part of your own dreams for your life. Once you stop building a life for others and start building your own, you'll find your life is filled with joy, beauty, and happiness. In short, you will be thriving.

To be truly successful at reclaiming your power and building the life of your dreams, you'll need to stop thinking of yourself as a victim. Remember, you are the hero of your own story. Your addicted spouse didn't happen to you, you're making the choice of your own free will to stay with him or her. Don't wait for your hero to arrive, be your own hero. You aren't a victim, you're the one making the decisions, and yes, taking the responsibility for those decisions. Only you can make yourself a victim. As your self-worth grows, you'll find you'll stop thinking of yourself in that way. You'll know and enforce your boundaries, you'll start truly writing your own story. You can achieve all of this regardless of who else is in your life. You have the power, you just have to claim it.

Relationships aren't easy, and when addiction enters the picture, it becomes even more complicated. However, addiction doesn't change the fact that you are in charge of your own life. You are writing your own story. By practicing many of the techniques we've discussed to set boundaries, boost your self-esteem, take charge of your own life, and take care of yourself, you'll start to truly transform your life. It will give you the strength to deal with the challenges you've accepted in your life. You'll learn to value your time and your choices so that you'll no longer sacrifice your needs for the desires of someone else. Your life will blossom and your choices will get easier. You'll be living life on your own terms, which everyone deserves to do.

JOURNAL ACTIVITY

For this journal activity, describe any ways in which you've given up your power in your relationship. Do you allow your spouse to make your decisions for you, or perhaps you always give in? Do you find you feel like you have to ask permission, or do you have trouble setting boundaries? Do you have problems with self-worth? What kinds of issues do you need to address to improve your self-worth? What can you do to take responsibility for your own life and become the author of your own story? Make a list of what you can do and make a commitment to implement at least one change a week for the next month. Keep track of the feelings that crop up as you do this activity. You'll often find that some challenging emotions arise as you go through this process.

As you work on increasing your self-worth, write about the boundaries you need to set in your relationship. Think about your values and desires and write down the kinds of boundaries that best define who you are as a person. Does your spouse regularly violate these boundaries? What can you do to set a firm boundary? What will be the consequences if your spouse violates a boundary you've set? Write out a strategy for what you will do to enforce those boundaries. Next, strategize how you will approach your spouse to express a need for these boundaries. By writing everything out, it helps ensure you don't forget what you might want to say, and it helps you organize your thoughts.

CHAPTER SUMMARY

In this chapter, we've discussed how to set strong boundaries and reclaim your power in the relationship you have with your addicted spouse. Specifically, we've covered the following topics:

- The importance of setting boundaries;
- The definition of a boundary;
- How a boundary reflects your values;
- How to set a boundary;
- What it looks like to lose power in a relationship;
- How to reclaim your power.

In the next chapter, you will learn some specific tips for taking care of yourself.

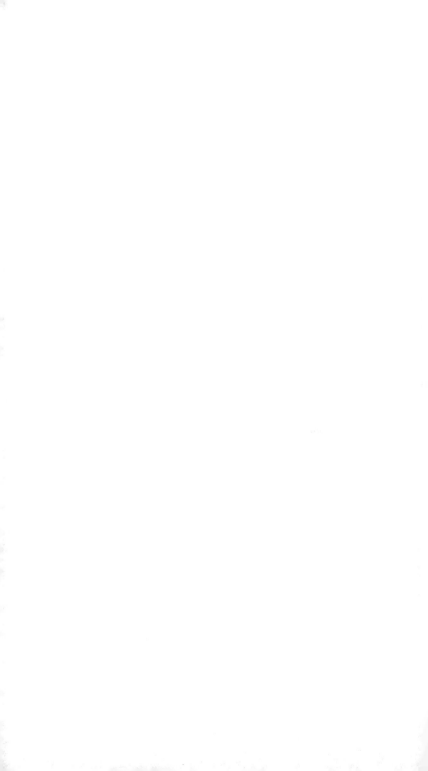

8

TAKING CARE OF YOU

IT's critical to take extra good care of yourself when you're involved with an addicted partner. Addicts are high maintenance in any relationship. As the spouse of an addict, you're most likely constantly worried about them. You might be afraid they won't come home one night because they got behind the wheel when they shouldn't have, or that they'll become angry when you bring up that you couldn't pay the phone bill because there wasn't enough money in the account. Perhaps you're most worried they'll never be able to overcome their addiction. You want them to be happy; yet, you're helpless to give them that sense of joy that can only come from within. When trying to help them beat their addiction and live a more productive life, it's easy to neglect yourself. By failing to take care of yourself, you only put yourself at risk for health problems, both mental and physical, and if something happens to you, who will take care of your family?

You begin the process of self-care by being mindful of your own needs. It's imperative to practice self-care every day.

Addiction is a family disease, and the spouse of an addict is on the front lines of a difficult battle. That can take a devastating emotional and physical toll. You feel the heartache of watching them sink further into a self-destructive spiral. You want to help them with their burden, and you might think that taking the time to practice daily self-care is something you just can't do. The reality is that if you don't do it, you'll sink into the depths of despair with them. That won't help anyone. So how can you take care of yourself? Let's look at some tips that can help.

CONSIDER INDIVIDUAL THERAPY

We've talked about letting go of feeling responsible for your addicted spouse's problems, but that can be very difficult to do. We've also talked about couples therapy and becoming involved in groups like codependency anonymous, but you might also need individual therapy to help you deal with the reasons behind why you feel so culpable for someone else's behavior. This can help you identify any issues you might need help to deal with, and it can help you to identify what is your "stuff" and what is your partner's "stuff." A therapist can also help you let go of what isn't yours to deal with. Individual therapy will help you alleviate your feelings of stress, anger, and pain associated with your partner's behavior. Having an objective therapist to talk to about your feelings can give you an enormous amount of relief. You'll find it is well worth your time.

TAKE CARE OF YOUR EMOTIONAL HEALTH

There are a number of ways in which you can boost your emotional health. Perhaps one of the most important is to cultivate and practice self-compassion. You're in a tough situation, and you need to recognize that sometimes you need to have compassion for yourself before you can have compassion for someone else. In fact, cultivating self-compassion will help you to feel compassion for your spouse.

One of the best ways to cultivate self-compassion is to imagine what you would say to your best friend if they told you they were going through what you are going through. It's likely you would feel a great deal of empathy for them. Why shouldn't you do the same for yourself? Try writing out what you would say to your friend in a journal and then read it to yourself. This can help you express your feelings as well as generate compassion for yourself.

Another way to take care of your emotional health is to practice mindfulness. Try the following exercise to help you explore your emotions and how they impact your body:

- Take a minimum of ten deep focused breaths.
- Now, focus on your body. How does it feel? Can you feel the cloth under your hands, the floor underneath your feet? Do you feel any areas of pain or stress? What do those feel like? Is the pain sharp or dull? Is it consistent or intermittent? Rather than trying to seek relief from the pain, take a moment to notice how it feels.
- Now, think of your addicted spouse. What do you notice? Do you feel something in your body? Does your breathing rate increase? What are the emotions you notice?
- Practice releasing the emotions from your body. Do this by visualizing your emotions lifting up from your body like smoke rising from an extinguished fire. Watch as the smoke wafts up and away from your body. Do this as many times as you need.

- Express gratitude for the life you've been given and for everything you have, including your addicted spouse. Recognize the opportunities in the challenges that lie before you and be grateful for the strength you have.
- Bring your focus back to your breath and take ten more deep belly-expanding breaths, and when you're ready, open your eyes.

Engaging in this type of mindfulness meditation will help you to realize when stress is affecting your body. It will help you to be mindful of your emotions as they arise, and that will help you to let them pass through your body. Letting them move through is key to preventing yourself from being traumatized by the situation. The important thing is to resist buying into the story that the emotions are telling you. They may be telling you something like, "you're so stupid," or "you don't deserve anything better." They may be weaving a tale of hopelessness. You can resist the urge to buy into that story by letting those emotions pass through you. You are a window through which the breeze of pain, fear, or disappointment passes. You experience the emotions, but you don't attach to them.

Another self-care technique ties into letting go of your emotions. It is to stay in the present moment. One of the things you notice the most when you stay in the present moment is that nothing is permanent. You might feel as though the feeling of despair will last forever, but if you stay present, you'll notice it isn't permanent. The intensity of the feeling fluctuates from moment to moment, and there are times when it isn't there at all. By staying in the present moment, you can also avoid catastrophizing about things that might happen in the future. Those things are not happening right now and staying in the present moment helps you keep from worrying. Worrying is a useless emotion. It has never saved anyone or prevented anything. It's like paying interest on a loan you might never get. It's damaging to your emotional health, and avoiding it will help you live a happier, more fulfilling life.

Another way to care for your emotional health is to get rid of that inner critic. We've briefly discussed replacing negative thoughts with positive ones, but it's such an important thing to do that it's worthwhile to elaborate on how to achieve that goal. One thing that is helpful to do is simply notice how many negative thoughts you have and when you tend to have them. They are like habits, after all, and replacing them with a good habit can be achieved with the same habit stacking practices discussed previously. First, however, you have to notice when you do it and why. Toward that end, try carrying a notebook around with you for a week, and just notice when you have a negative thought. Write down the thought you had as well as what preceded it, what kinds of emotions accompanied the thought, and any additional feelings or thoughts that occurred as a result of the self-criticism. It's also helpful to notice who else was present when you had the thought.

At the end of the week, you will have a list of the negative thoughts you typically have, as well as the triggers that caused them. The next step is to replace each negative thought with a positive affirmation. If you tend to think, "I'm so stupid," when you catch your addicted spouse in a lie, replace that with, "I am growing in compassion and forgiveness for my spouse." If you tend to think, "I don't deserve any better," replace that with, "I am lovingly expressing my self-worth." Write each of these positive affirmations down and carry that list with you. Each time you find yourself thinking one of

those negative thoughts, pull out your sheet of positive affirmations and read your replacement out loud to yourself. Just
like the habit stacking discussed earlier, these positive
thoughts will start to become the habit in place of negative
thoughts. As this happens, you'll start to notice considerable
improvements in your mood.

LET GO OF REGRET

It's common for the spouse of an addict to feel regret for
things they may have done that added to the problem or
mistakes they have made in the past. They commonly feel
shame associated with these feelings. Just like worry, shame
and guilt are useless emotions. You can't go back in time and
undo something you have done, and everyone makes
mistakes. The fact that you are ashamed of something you
did just goes to show you that you are not the same person
now as you were then. You've grown and changed, and so
you resolve to make better choices for your behavior in the
future. Again, practice that mindfulness meditation to let go
of those useless feelings. You can't change what you did in the
past, but you can change how you react now. That's what
you're doing, so let go of those old feelings, stop living in the
past, and stay grounded in the present.

It's also common to feel shame for your addicted spouse's
actions. The combination of his or her feelings, experiences,
or actions with your own can make the situation extremely
intense and uncomfortable. You might find yourself thinking
thoughts like, "I can't believe you're choosing alcohol over
me," or "You are a disgrace to our family," and those
thoughts are often followed by feelings of anger, shame, or
disappointment. This is a good time to practice that self-
compassion discussed previously. Of course you have those

kinds of feelings in that situation. Who wouldn't? Accept those emotions and let them pass through you. Acknowledge that things are not ideal and that people you love are suffering. If you fall into the trap of believing that things are supposed to be a certain way instead of accepting how things are, you'll be at risk of feeling isolated and culpable.

Don't be afraid to ask for help from your community and people who are going through the same thing. You are not alone, and the situation is not your fault. Talking to other people going through the same thing can help you understand that and support you as you seek to help your addicted spouse.

WRITE YOURSELF A LOVE LETTER

There's nothing like a love letter to pick up your day. It's also a nice way to practice some self-love. Write yourself a love letter admiring all of your best qualities. You're not bragging, you're being honest. You're strong, patient, loving, and kind. Tell yourself that in the same way you would tell a lover. Be warm, gentle, and loving to yourself. When you're done writing it, put it in an envelope, address it, and put a stamp on it. After that, give it to a friend and ask them to drop it in the mail sometime in the next month. Ask them not to tell you when they've done that, and that way, it will be a surprise when you get it. It's sure to bring a smile to your face.

PLAY LIKE A CHILD

Do you remember when you would lay in the grass of summer and watch the clouds go by? Do you remember running and laughing and playing as if you didn't have a care in the world? Enjoying the sweet smell of cut grass, the long, sunny days, feeling like everything was right with the world? Just because you're an adult now doesn't mean you should stop playing. Play like you did during those carefree days. Dance around your house as if no one is watching, sing at the top of your lungs, run through an open field, or lay on the grass and watch the clouds go by. In short, find something carefree that makes you feel as joyful as you did way back then, and do it at least once a week, if not every day. Let go of your worries for a few carefree hours and lose yourself in something you're passionate about, something that brings you unmitigated joy. You'll feel better and that will make you treat everyone in your life better. Your mind will be clearer, your emotions will be more positive, and your energy will soar.

A FEW OF YOUR FAVORITE THINGS

Entertain your favorite things to do. That might mean spending the day at the spa, going out with your friends, fishing, camping, or hiking. Go for a run, take yourself out to a movie you've been wanting to see, or go stargazing. This is part of self-care. Make the time to do the things you enjoy every week and do a little something every day. Doing something you enjoy will refresh your mind, energize your body, and lighten your soul.

GET HEALTHY

One of the best things you can do for yourself when living with someone afflicted with addiction is to get and stay healthy. You're going through a lot of stressful situations that take a toll on your physical health. You have to take extra care to ensure you stay physically healthy. To do that, you have to recognize your own needs and prioritize time to attend to them. Your needs are just as important as your partner's, and they deserve your attention as well. Being a strong partner means you have to be in good physical and mental health. If you are going to help your partner through a healing process, you'll need to be prepared for a marathon, which means taking care of your physical, mental, and spiritual needs.

We've discussed the importance of mindfulness meditation and seeking individual therapy to help care for your emotional and mental needs. These are critical for helping you deal with the many difficult emotions you face on a daily basis. There are, however, more tips that can help.

Spiritual rituals: Whatever kind of spirituality you practice (if any), make sure to take some time each day to engage in the important rituals of your faith. Faith can bolster your sense of purpose and self-worth. If you're an atheist or agnostic, practicing meditation can give you the same kind of satisfaction--no faith required, just quiet your mind and let yourself be free of your worries for a little while.

Find someone positive to interact with each day: Positive people make you feel positive about yourself and your own potential. Find someone who can help you bolster your self-esteem and you'll feel better about yourself, which will improve your interactions with everyone else in your life.

Exercise: You need to take time to exercise regularly. Exercise produces endorphins in the brain, and those make you feel better about the world. Furthermore, exercise is a proven way to reduce anxiety, stress, and depression. This is exactly what you need if you're taking care of an addicted spouse. You might think you don't have time, but you can start with a mere fifteen to twenty minutes of exercise each day and work up to longer periods as time allows. It will help you keep your head clear and your body strong.

Get enough sleep: Sleep is essential to good health. If you don't get enough sleep or if the quality of your sleep is not good, it can leave you feeling exhausted and like you can't think straight. If you're having trouble getting good sleep, the following tips will help:

- Keep your bedroom dark, cool, and quiet.
- Don't watch TV or use your cell phone or computer right before bed--the blue light from the screens interferes with good sleep.
- Listen to relaxing music before bed.
- Use white noise or soothing natural sounds like rain gently falling or waves lapping at the shore as background noise to help you sleep.
- Drink a cup of caffeine-free tea.
- Meditate right before bed.
- Take a hot bath with Epsom salts.
- Practice deep breathing--the kind that expands your belly--before going to bed. This type of breathing activates the vagus nerve, which turns on your parasympathetic nervous system. The parasympathetic nervous system is otherwise known as the "relax and chill" nervous system. It calms your body down, and that's how deep breathing can help relax you.

Make healthy food choices: Eating healthy will keep your body functioning properly and help you avoid becoming sick. Eat plenty of antioxidant-rich foods, make sure you get enough vitamins and minerals in your diet, and eat some antidepressant foods like dark chocolate to keep you in a positive mood.

Keep your children in a positive mindset: Another thing that can help you stay positive is if you also keep your children in a positive mindset. It's important that you not turn to them for support since they've got enough on their plate just being kids. You also want them to have a positive view of their other parent, even though that parent might be currently addicted to drugs or alcohol. Of course, you should keep them safe from physical or emotional abuse perpetrated by your addicted spouse, but you should strive to keep them out of it as much as possible. They should understand their other parent is sick, and that can make them act out sometimes, but they still love them. You want them to have as stable a life as possible since enduring an addicted parent during childhood can have many negative effects that last long into adulthood.

By following these tips for taking care of yourself and your family, it will help you keep a positive outlook on your situation. It's important that you take good care of yourself since you are the one bearing the lion's share of the responsibility for caring for the rest of the family. It's also important to keep in mind that taking care of yourself means much more than simply taking care of your physical health. You also need to attend to your spiritual, emotional, and mental needs.

JOURNAL ACTIVITY

For this journal activity, you're going to practice some healthy self-care. First, write down the things you need to do to take better care of yourself and how you can make those a reality. It might mean going to bed earlier so you can get a better night's sleep, or it might mean getting up a few minutes earlier so you can get in fifteen minutes of exercise. List at least two things you can start in the next week to begin taking better care of yourself.

Next, write out something for which you feel regret. It might be something related to an interaction with your addicted spouse or it could be an older wound. Let go of the shame you feel around that incident. Practice the mindfulness meditation where you visualize the painful feelings as drifting out of your body like smoke rising from an extinguished fire. Record your feelings about what you've experienced.

Finally, write down two childhood memories you have of playing in a carefree manner. What were you doing? Who were you with? Is it something you can do now or can you do something similar? Make a plan to play a little each day for the next week and record your feelings about it after you give yourself the gift of play.

CHAPTER SUMMARY

In this chapter, we've discussed the importance of taking care of yourself. Specifically, we've discussed the following topics:

- Why it might be a good idea to consider individual therapy;
- The importance of taking care of your emotional needs;
- Attending to your spiritual needs;
- Taking care of your physical health;
- Taking care of your children so you'll be happier.

In the next chapter, you'll learn about how to create the reality you want with the power of your mind.

9

CREATING YOUR HIGHEST GOOD

WHEN YOU'VE REGAINED your self-confidence, improved your self-esteem, and taken back some of your personal power, it's possible to take an active role in creating the reality you want to see in your life. In each of us, there is greatness, and you can use that to consciously direct your mind and your life. Once you understand the true nature of reality, you can use the laws of the universe to bring abundance, love, and happiness into your life. You are a powerful co-creator with direct access to the divine universal energy, and you can use it to bring goodness into your reality. You can't force change on your addicted partner, but you can lead by example, something which might inspire change in your loved ones, too. Let's look at how this works.

HIGHER CONSCIOUSNESS

There is a part of you, the observer inside, that is aware of the fact that the physical world--what you think of as reality--is only an illusion. It is, as Einstein said, "A very persistent one," but it is an illusion, nonetheless. Your circumstances represent a reflection of your inner world, and your inner world is simply a product of your thoughts. Thus, if you change your thoughts, you will change your circumstances. Your higher consciousness, that part of you that observes, knows this is true. It is now, and always remains, at peace, because it is your connection to the one universal mind. No matter the chaos in your life, it is the part of you that is never disturbed by anything. It's the part of you that knows this is but a dream. Moreover, this higher consciousness cannot be subjected to negative programming, something that distinguishes it from your subconscious mind. To access this peaceful, fearless part of you, you only have to become aware of it. That's all, nothing more.

To become aware of your higher consciousness, the next time you feel an emotion, instead of focusing your attention on the emotion, try focusing your attention on the part of you that is aware of or noticing the emotion. That's your higher consciousness, that's the real you. When you can access this higher consciousness regularly, you'll find that you can accept what appears to be reality without judgment or fear, and you can begin to direct the course of your life to create circumstances that are preferable to you. You begin to fully access your higher consciousness by deciding to allow only empowering, positive, and nurturing messages to enter your conscious mind. You notice immediately when a negative thought attempts to enter, and you simply stop it and replace it with a positive message, something that will empower the change you want to see in your life. With time, you'll find that fewer and fewer negative messages even try to enter the realm of your conscious mind.

Once your higher consciousness is running the show, you can now use techniques such as creative visualization and meditation to open yourself up to a world of miracles wherein you can consciously create your own reality. In essence you're using three parts of your mind; your subconscious, which can't reason (it only reacts); your conscious mind, which is reason; and your higher consciousness, which doesn't need to reason; to create any kind of circumstances you want to have in your life. You've already been using your subconscious and conscious minds in this way, and the fear and anxiety you're experiencing in your current reality reflects the fear and anxiety that runs rampant in those realms when the higher consciousness is not in charge. When you put your higher consciousness at the helm, you can create a heaven on earth for yourself. This higher consciousness is even referenced in the Bible. It is what Jesus Christ meant when he said, "The kingdom of heaven is within." It truly is within you, and it is within your ability to miraculously transform your life. One of the powerful ways to do this is with creative visualization.

CREATIVE VISUALIZATION

This is the fundamental technique for creating your own reality. You are using your thoughts to consciously imagine what you want to create in your life. When you do that, you create and attract into your life exactly what you need to realize your ideal life. This gives you direct control over your subconscious mind, and when you program your subconscious mind, it summons the ideas and emotions that get results fast. Your subconscious mind has already been generating your reality, but instead of you consciously directing it to create what you want, your fears and insecurities have been directing it to bring the things you don't want into your life. Your negative thoughts were the seeds to bring your greatest fears to life. Now, you'll plant seeds of abundance, joy, and love, and those will be drawn into your reality using this technique.

There are five basic steps that you can use to visualize your intentions in order to create your ideal reality. The five steps are: relax, imagine, feel, believe, and detach. Let's take a closer look:

Step 1: Relax

If you want to relax your body, you have to relax your mind. To do that, find a comfortable seat and sit upright while breathing deeply and steadily. Count down slowly from 25 to 1 while at the same time, relaxing your muscle groups starting at your head and progressing down your body to your toes. Focus on your breath to empty your mind.

Step 2: Imagine

The next step is to imagine your intended outcome. Your imagination is the engine for your thoughts, and it has the power to convert them into mental images. Imagine your reality in the present moment. Pretend you're watching a movie, but one in which you're the star. As you watch your life unfolding exactly how you want it to, concentrate on what you're seeing, hearing, feeling, and experiencing in all its richness. Focus on indulging your senses fully.

Step 3: Feel

The next step is to feel what it would be like if you already had what you want. This means really feel it. For example, if you envisioned that you're getting a promotion, let yourself feel your jubilation at that reality. If you envisioned that you're renewing your wedding vows with your now addiction-free spouse, let yourself feel the love and joy as if it were happening right now. While your imagination is the engine for your thoughts, your feelings are the fuel for that engine. Your emotions are energy in action, they bring your images to life.

Step 4: Believe

The next step is to believe that you already have what you intend to have, right now, in the present moment. This isn't about lying to yourself or even just wishful thinking, it's about knowing the truth behind creating your own reality. It's about having faith in the evidence of things you can't see. The idea is that by believing you already have what you've imagined you'll have, you'll act in a way that is consistent with someone who has those things, and then they will become your reality. This works, so take a leap of faith and believe. You'll be amazed at what happens.

Step 5: Detach

This is an extremely important step. The process of creative visualization works, but sometimes it works in ways you don't anticipate. That's why it's vital to detach from a specific outcome. You might have a very specific intention, but if you place constraints on the outcome by becoming attached to it playing out in a set way, you effectively strip yourself of your authentic power to create the life you want to live. You will succeed in creating your ideal life, but you need to let the universe work its magic. It will bring into your life precisely what you need to achieve your intended goals, but it may do that in creative ways.

What this means is that it isn't like asking Santa Claus for a bicycle. You're not asking God or the universe to give you A, B, or C. What you want to imagine and intend when creating your reality are the general outcomes--abundance, love, joy. Abundance, for example, can be achieved in a number of ways. You might get to the abundance you desire because you get that promotion you want, or the universe might work it so that you lose that job, but find one that pays much better. If you creatively visualize your spouse as being addiction-free and the two of you renewing your wedding vows, your spouse might decide to seek help for his or her addiction, but they might have to sink to rock bottom before they make that decision. What you intend to create might not always unfold in the most obvious way, so if you detach yourself from specific outcomes and instead set overall goals, you'll be better able to see the opportunities unfolding as the universe works to bring your ideal life into your reality.

So visualize the outcomes you desire in terms of the feelings or other things it will bring you. Abundance would allow you to buy your dream house, and therefore, visualize yourself in your dream house as if you have it right now. If your spouse is addiction-free, your life will be dramatically different. Visualize exactly how it will be different as if it is right now. You and your spouse are communicating easily, doing things together, and loving each other fully. What you're not visualizing in either of these examples, however, is exactly how you got to that point. That's where the universe will surprise you.

You effectively detach by leaving the "how" up to the universe. Focus on the outcome, which is your happy life with your addiction-free spouse, rather than on the process. Release any control regarding how your ideal life will be achieved. Once you've visualized your ideal life, say to the universe, "I leave the specifics to you."

When you've completed this visualization process, you can return to your normal waking state. Count from 1 to 5 to bring yourself out of your relaxed state and slowly open your eyes. If you're doing this visualization at night, you can let yourself drift off to sleep.

Practice

It's important to practice creative visualization frequently. In fact, it's ideal to practice the technique when you wake up to set the best intentions for your day and before you go to sleep to set the intentions firmly in your subconscious mind so it can work while you sleep. Practicing regularly will bring you the best and most rapid results. You'll begin to see your life transforming in ways you never thought possible.

Inspired Action

You also want to follow up your creative visualization practices with inspired action. This means you want to be calm and deliberate in the actions you take. You want to listen to your intuition and look for those opportunities the universe brings your way. If you do lose that job, for example, instead of thinking that your visualizations didn't work, look for the opportunity that is being presented to you. You now can look for a better paying job or pursue your dream career. If you see that your spouse seems to be sinking deeper into addiction, understand that the opportunity in that situation is for them to finally hit rock bottom and decide to make healthy changes. Stand your ground on your boundaries, stay true to yourself, and that might finally make your spouse see that they need to change. If not, then maybe it's time to leave, but do so with the understanding that you're not trying to punish them, but to save yourself. Do so with the understanding that the universe is working to bring your ideal life into your reality. You may not see it clearly at the moment, but keep the faith and keep looking for those opportunities. If you do so, you will find your ideal life.

CHAPTER SUMMARY

In this chapter, we've discussed the technique of creative visualization to use the power of your mind to create your ideal life. Specifically, we've covered the following topics:

- The role of your higher consciousness in creating your ideal life;
- Programming your subconscious mind to work for you instead of against you;
- The definition and steps for creative visualization;
- The importance of regularly practicing creative visualization;
- Letting the universe work out the details.

The next chapter will present some final words.

FINAL WORDS

There's no more difficult relationship than one in which you watch the person you love engage in self-destructive behavior. It's hard to understand why they wouldn't simply stop this behavior, but the reality is they are dealing with a brain disease. They are quite literally hardwired to crave their favorite substance. Furthermore, it's not your responsibility to fix your spouse. The only way they can get better is if they choose to heal themselves. Does that mean that you can't stay in your relationship? No, you can stay in your relationship, but it will take a lot of work on your part.

You'll need to stay mindful of your feelings and needs, and you'll need to ensure that your needs are met. Your addicted spouse will not be capable of taking care of your needs. It's not that they don't love you, it's that they're not capable of focusing on anything other than their addiction. There's no doubt that if your spouse is not in some kind of recovery, you're choosing a very difficult road for yourself. You'll need a healthy dose of self-confidence and strong boundaries.

You'll also need to be clear and honest in your communications with your partner. You'll want to ensure that the environment where you and your children live is safe and free of drugs and alcohol. You may have to refrain from the occasional glass of wine you might enjoy if it will trigger the craving in your spouse. There will be a lot of sacrifice on your part, which is why it's essential you take good care of yourself. You'll need to practice regular, high quality self-care. Take an occasional spa day or go camping with friends. Meditate, play every day, spend time doing things you like to do, and exercise. You'll need your health and stamina to keep going through what can become some very difficult challenges.

It's helpful to remember that if you stay grounded in the present moment, it will be easier to see through the addiction to the loving soul inside the addict. When you can do that, you'll be better able to communicate your needs in a sensitive, honest, and clear manner that will get better results. Addiction is also a family disease, and it will be helpful to work on the issues together as a family. For that to happen, you have to accept your partner as is, without wanting to change him or her. You can only help yourself, and working together to set boundaries and improve communication and respect for each other, will produce better results than going it alone.

To maintain your own healthy self-esteem and confidence, you might also have to face some of your own demons. There are many ways to do that, but a big part of your own healing is accepting the shadow parts of yourself that feel aggrieved with each slight to your ego. These are the parts of you that were hurt long ago when you didn't get the healing, loving response you needed from those closest to you at that time. Welcome them back into the whole you to help heal yourself from those old traumas. The whole you will be better at supporting your addicted partner through their pain, and the whole you will be better able to practice good self-care.

If you adhere to these tips, your relationship could last through an eventual recovery, and if that never comes, you'll be able to create a safe environment where you can still grow professionally, personally, and spiritually. You can't save your partner, only they can do that. You have to save yourself, and you have to be your own priority. Use this book as your guide to help you on this difficult journey. Use your journal as a written plan for understanding your feelings, deciding what you need, and strategizing on how you will implement the changes you want to see in your life.

Let's end the beginning of your new journey with some creative visualization:

(Play relaxing music)

- Sit in a relaxed position but one in which you won't fall asleep.
- Close your eyes and focus on your breath. Notice how it flows in through your nose to expand your chest. Allow it also to expand your belly. Feel the air filling your lungs and then follow it as it exits through your nose. Take ten deep belly-expanding breaths while staying focused.
- Imagine that each time you inhale, you're breathing in relaxation. Now, with each exhale you're breathing out tension. As you continue breathing exhale forcefully through your mouth to expel tension. Take ten breaths in this manner--inhale relaxation through your nose, exhale tension forcefully through your mouth.
- Breathe slowly and gently now.

- Continue to take calm breaths as you focus on relaxing your body. Notice how each area of your body mentioned relaxes as soon as you hear the word "relax."
- Focus on your head... relax…
- Focus on your face.... relax…
- Now, your neck.... relax…
- Your shoulders... relax
- Your upper arms… relax...
- Your lower arms… relax…
- Your hands and fingers… relax…
- Your chest… relax…
- Your abdomen… relax…
- Your hips… relax…
- Your pelvis… relax…
- Your bottom… relax…
- Your upper legs… relax…
- Your lower legs… relax…
- Your feet and toes… relax...
- Scan your body now for any remaining areas of tension and focus your attention on these areas while relaxing them more.
- Now that your body has started to become relaxed, with each breath in, say in your mind, "breathe."
- With each breath out, mentally say, "relax."
- Move your focus to your body. How does it feel? What do your hands feel like resting on your lap or legs? Can you feel the cloth of your pants against your skin? Can you feel your shoes on your feet? Take inventory of your body, noticing all the sensations you are experiencing.
- Turn your focus to your life. Imagine what your life would look like if you got everything you wanted. Your spouse is free from his or her addiction, and

your love has blossomed. What does that look like? How does a typical day go? Don't just envision it, but feel what it's like to have your spouse expressing their love for you, feel what it's like to be experiencing life together. Let yourself feel those feelings as if all of that were true right now. How does it feel to have your bills paid off? Feel what it's like as if it is true in the present moment. Imagine every aspect of your life that you want to improve and let the feeling of success flow through your body. Let those feelings flood your body.

- Express gratitude for what you have. See the gratitude in you as a golden white light in your heart space. Envision the light spreading to the rest of your body. Express gratitude for your health, your sound mind, home, and family. Let the light spread beyond the bounds of your body. Express gratitude for your neighborhood, your friends, and extended family, then let it spread to your broader community. Express gratitude for your city, your state, your country. See the golden white light bathing everything in gratitude. Now, let it spread to the planet, and then, the universe. Give thanks for your life and the opportunity to rise above the challenges you face.
- Now, bring your focus back to your breath. Take ten more belly-expanding breaths.
- Open your eyes when you feel you're ready.

This is an excellent meditation to practice every morning and every evening.

When you've finished this meditation, write in your journal about the feelings you experienced as you envisioned your perfect life. Complete the following sentence in your journal no less than ten times: "My life will be ideal when..." Once you've identified the goals you want to achieve, the next step will be to set a few milestones that will move you closer to achieving between one and three of those goals. Taking action will empower you and practicing visualizing meditation regularly will keep you motivated and help you relieve any stress and anxiety you may be feeling. Remember that you deserve good things in life, you deserve love, and you deserve respect. You deserve to realize your perfect life. It can be done. It takes developing self-love, expressing gratitude for what you have, realizing what your baggage is and what belongs to your spouse, and letting go of what you can't control. You are worthwhile so it's time to convince yourself of that and start truly living your life. You deserve every good thing that comes your way, so go get it!

ABOUT THE AUTHOR

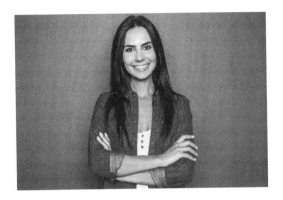

Dhana Raphael Michaels has been an advocate for the millions of families impacted by addiction for many years. As both the wife of an alcoholic and the mother of an alcoholic, Dhana has experienced firsthand the devastating effects of addiction on families.

Dhana has dedicated her life to helping other families dealing with this disease, compiling everything she has learned through her own personal process and everything she knows from her professional pursuits -- combining them here and delivered in the hope that she might be able to ease some of your own pain and suffering. Dhana currently lives in New York City, where she raises her five-year-old grandchild on her own. In her free time, she enjoys painting and journaling.

You can find out more about her work at www.GoodFortuneWorldWide.com.

Sobriety Journal

Made in the USA
Middletown, DE
13 November 2020